RESEARCH HIGHLIGHTS IN SOCIAL WORK 31

Dementia: Challenges and New Directions

Faith in
Older People

Registered Charity SC038225
Registered Company SC322915

21a Grosvenor Crescent
EDINBURGH EH12 5EL
Tel: 0131 346 7981

Email: info@fiop.org.uk
Website: fiop@dioceseofedinburgh.org

Developing Services for Older People and their Families
Edited by Rosemary Bland
ISBN 1 85302 290 X

Past Trauma in Late Life
European Perspectives on Therapeutic Work with Older People
Edited by Linda Hunt, Mary Marshall and Cherry Rowlings
ISBN 1 85302 446 5

Hearing the Voice of People with Dementia
Opportunities and Obstacles
Malcolm Goldsmith
ISBN 1 85302 406 6

Dementia
New Skills for Social Workers
Edited by Alan Chapman and Mary Marshall
ISBN 1 85302 142 3

Reviewing Care Management for Older People
Edited by Judith Phillips and Bridget Penhale
ISBN 1 85302 317 5

RESEARCH HIGHLIGHTS IN SOCIAL WORK 31

Dementia: Challenges and New Directions

Edited by Susan Hunter

Jessica Kingsley Publishers
London and Bristol, Pennsylvania

Robert Gordon University
School of Applied Social Studies
Kepplestone Annexe, Queen's Road
Aberdeen AB9 2PG

All rights reserved. No paragraph of this publication may be reproduced, copied or trans-
mitted save with written permission or in accordance with the provisions of the Copyright Act 1956 (as amended), or under the terms of any licence permitting limited
copying issued by the Copyright Licensing Agency, 33–34 Alfred Place, London WC1E
7DP. Any person who does any unauthorised act in relation to this publication may be liable to criminal prosecution and civil claims for damages.

The right of the contributors to be identified as author of this work has been asserted by
them in accordance with the Copyright, Designs and Patents Act 1988.

First published in the United Kingdom in 1997 by
Jessica Kingsley Publishers Ltd
116 Pentonville Road
London N1 9JB, England
and
1900 Frost Road, Suite 101
Bristol, PA 19007, U S A

Copyright © 1997 Robert Gordon University, Research Highlights Advisory Group,
School of Applied Social Studies

Library of Congress Cataloging in Publication Data
A CIP catalogue record for this book is available from the Library of Congress

British Library Cataloguing in Publication Data
Social work with people with dementia – (Research highlights in social work; 31)
  1. Dementia 2. Mentally Ill – Care 3. Mental health services
  I. Hunter, Susan
  362.2

ISBN 1 85302 312 4

Printed and Bound in Great Britain by
Athenæum Press, Gateshead, Tyne and Wear

Contents

Part III: User And Carer Perspectives

Part IV: Service Provision Issues

List of tables

List of figures

Introduction

Susan Hunter

This is the first volume in the Research Highlights series to be devoted exclusively to dementia. Perhaps this is a reflection of the transformation in dementia's status from a topic of relative neglect to one of increasing interest in all domains of our society, be they professional, public or political. There are some well-rehearsed explanations for this burgeoning interest, some of which will be developed in this volume and some of which will be challenged by it. In particular this study seeks to refocus the agenda to take account of the positive vision and encouraging achievements of a new generation of researchers and practitioners and away from the negativism which has characterised so much writing on dementia in the past.

Some urgency is being brought to bear on the task of incorporating new information and ideas into our services by the rapidly changing environment in which we operate. Increased professional awareness and advances in diagnostic expertise will mean that increasing numbers of people with dementia and their carers will be brought into the service net, over and above those resulting from the predicted expansion in the highest risk age groups. Improved public understanding of, and empathy for, dementia sufferers and consequent reductions in the stigma attached to the condition will combine with legislative initiatives such as the Carers Services and Recognition Act (1995) to reinforce the legitimacy of both user and carer demands and requirements. The pressures which will be brought to bear on services by the promotion of the mixed economy of welfare are particularly complex in the field of dementia as it attempts to find ways in which the service users and their carers can fulfil the aspirations of the NHS and Community Care Act (1990) as consumers in the welfare 'supermarket' and as partners in decision-making about their care. The exercise of choice, and particularly informed choice, in a service provision arena which is destined to become increasingly diverse, poses a serious challenge to services further complicated by the loss of resources within the NHS.

Editorial selectivity is inevitable in a work dealing with a field as vast as that of dementia, but it has been exercised with this new agenda in mind. The book is divided into four parts, each of which attempts to reflect and explore the changing agenda in specific ways.

Section 1: Context

This opening section, which aims to set the context for this volume, deliberately starts with a challenge to orthodox models for understanding of dementia which are based largely on neuropathology. Kitwood explores the concept of personhood and the ground-breaking possibilities its practical applications offer in the management of dementia. This 'new humanism', as he terms it, is of course replete with the ethical dilemmas and pitfalls so vividly set out in Alan Jacques' chapter which underscores the complexities of substitute decision-making whether by carers, by professionals or by the law. In this context it becomes critical to preserve individual autonomy and capacity for as long as possible by utilising the enhanced clinical and care expertise described later in the volume.

Exceptionally for a text on dementia, the reader will not find a classic account of the nature and incidence of the condition. This is well documented in other places (Jacques 1992). In the discussion of demography, Gordon and Spicker throw down a gauntlet that the figures are, 'hardly likely to bring the collapse of civilisation as we know it' and suggest the real challenge lies not in meeting accumulated individual need but in devising a strategy for gathering information which is 'future-proofed', that is, capable of responding to the needs of future cohorts which can be predicted to be quite different from those of the current generation.

Section 2: Selected aspects of dementia

The three chapters in the second section all focus on aspects of dementia which traditionally have not been mainstream concerns but which have emerged as significant issues in their own right as our knowledge base has expanded and become more sophisticated. They examine ways in which evolving knowledge, whilst opening up new possibilities for treatment and for the development of supportive services, can also create new ethical dilemmas. Whalley alerts us to the profound challenges which arise out of advances in knowledge of the genetic, environmental and disease-related contributions to early onset dementia, together with the implications for risk prediction and the use of therapeutic genes. Warrington's chapter, whilst acknowledging the progress made in differentiating depression and dementia, points to the dangers for individuals of the lack of understanding of the co-existence of these two conditions which, if unrecognised and untreated, further undermines their ability to function. Similarly Holland points to the compelling evidence that people with Down's syndrome are 'at particular risk' of developing Alzheimer's dementia, but warns against the automatic assumption that either is the cause of any deterioration when there could be other treatable causes.

The recurring theme of these three chapters is the nature of the challenge of ensuring that treatable conditions do not go untreated and that management implications are taken on board in order to avoid further undermining of individual integrity.

Section 3: User and carer perspectives

Consultation with those who depend on services and their carers has become one of the major currencies of community care activity. The chapters in Section 3 reveal just how far conventional wisdom and practice are lagging behind current knowledge and understanding. Based on his own work and a few existing studies, Goldsmith demonstrates that the voice of people with dementia can, and should, be heard, and discusses what needs to change in order to make services and attitudes more inclusive. Parker's chapter sets out for our consideration the complexities, professional and ethical, of assessing carer stress and providing services to alleviate that stress in ways which are effective, equitable and transparent. We are reminded that there is little agreement about the relationship between these stresses and the degree of carer stress. The chapter goes on to explore how there may be a mismatch, at least in relation to dementia, between the orthodoxy of targeting scarce resources through 'objective' assessment of dependency and the research which suggests that stress is mediated through far more subjective factors.

Section 4: Service provision issues

The final section contains discussion of four areas in service provision which are ripe for consideration and in which developments are moving apace. Public attitudes towards care in the community for people with dementia are known to be less favourable than towards other community care groups (West, Illsley and Kelman 1984). So knowledge about the ways in which people with dementia can be successfully supported in the community assumes particular importance. This account by Challis and colleagues of the findings of an intensive care management experiment suggests, contrary to some previous research, that care management can improve the outcomes for people with dementia and their carers.

A 'significant minority' of people with dementia live in long-stay institutional settings where maintenance of quality of life can be hazardous for people whose capacity to speak up for themselves may be diminished (p.165). The next two chapters, by Gilloran and Downs and by Marshall, constitute two sides of the same coin. They explore two important strands in the development of positive social care environments. Gilloran and Downs draw attention to the crucial role of staff morale in being able to exploit the rapidly expanding range of therapies and activities now available to support an improved quality of life. Marshall, on the other hand, explores factors in the built environment and its design which can be harnessed to maximise the autonomy of individuals. Central to her argument is the idea of dementia as a disability, i.e. as something more than the complex illness it undoubtedly is. Drawing from the design literature and practice accounts she offers both the inspiration and the practical advice for challenging the 'fundamental lack of belief' that design should be taken seriously as a factor in therapeutic care.

The final chapter describes the evolution of independent advocacy and why it is increasingly important in our changing world. At the heart of Burton's chapter lies the profound challenge of safeguarding – safeguarding the rights of people with dementia. As she and other contributors remind us, the law in this area is obsolete and pending overhaul, while families and service professionals are often called upon to face conflicts of interest in the decision-making process. Notwithstanding the complexities of using a 'substituted judgement' approach, Burton's own small study highlights the potential effectiveness of advocacy in achieving greater participation in decision-making and greater access to resources so that, 'dementia sufferers are placed at the heart of the decision-making process and that their voice is both heard and respected'.

Those readers interested in up-to-date accounts of the developments in day care and what, for convenience, is called 'respite care' are directed to companion volumes in this series (Bland 1996; Stalker 1996). Also valuable work which should attract attention in the future has been undertaken in two areas, namely the development of dementia services for ethnic minorities (see Brownlie 1991 and Manthorpe and Hettiaratchy 1993) and of frameworks for the management by others of vulnerable individuals' finances (see Langan and Means 1995).

Concluding comments

This volume has attempted to set out some of the challenges and new directions in the field of dementia studies. We seem to be moving from an era of relative neglect, in which dementia services were truly the Cinderella among adult care services, to one which offers opportunities for radical and positive development. The following themes are emerging as the focal points for these future developments:

- the overhaul and modernisation of the legal and ethical frameworks within which services operate

- the creation of therapeutic optimism based on inclusion and holistic approaches to the study of dementia, in part inspired by the insights offered by a new generation of researchers

- the increasingly robust articulation of the user and carer voice.

It is arguable that all this constitutes a 'paradigm shift', to use a term from a writer in another field (Kinsella 1992). Insofar as a paradigm is a set of concepts governing a world view, a shift in these concepts implies a complete conceptual revolution which in turn changes all established practices and conventions. We are now on the threshold of such a shift and it is hoped that this modest publication will play its part in heralding in the new era of dementia care and provide some markers on the way.

Acknowledgements

I would like to thank Joyce Lishman and the editorial advisory committee for their support in realising this project, Anne Forbes for her precision typing and Mary Marshall for some well-timed comments. Not least of all, I'm grateful to all the authors who took time out of busy schedules to contribute so willingly and generously to this volume.

References

Bland, R. (1996) *Developing Services for Older People and their Families*. London: Jessica Kingsley Publishers.

Brownlie, J. (1991) *A Hidden Problem? Dementia Amongst Minority Ethnic Groups*. Stirling: University of Stirling, Dementia Services Development Centre.

Jacques, A. (1992) *Understanding Dementia*. Edinburgh: Churchill Livingstone.

Kinsella, P. (1992) *Shifting Mountains...Shifting Paradigms*. New York: Harkness Fellow, The Commonwealth Fund of New York.

Langan, J. and Means, R. (1995) *Personal Finances, Elderly People with Dementia and the New Community Care*. Research Report no.8. Kidlington: Anchor Housing Association.

Manthorpe, J. and Hettiaratchy, P. (1993) 'Ethnic minority elders in the UK.' *International Review of Psychiatry 5*, 171–178.

Stalker, K. (1996) *Developments in Short-Term Care: Breaks and Opportunities*. London: Jessica Kingsley Publishers.

West, P., Illsley, R. and Kelman, H. (1984) 'Public preferences for the care of dependence groups.' *Social Science and Medicine 18*, 287–298.

PART I
Context

Chapter 1

Personhood, Dementia and Dementia Care

Tom Kitwood

As the twentieth century draws towards its close, the industrialised societies of the western world find themselves in an extraordinary and paradoxical predicament. It is becoming clear that the system of liberal democracy, the economic life of which is grounded in the pursuit of profit, is incapable of delivering a secure and prosperous way of life for all its citizens. In many nation states 'welfare capitalism' is virtually at an end. And yet, even while old expectations have been breaking down, a new culture of caring has been gaining ground; more strongly committed, more psychologically aware, more practical and more pragmatic than anything that has gone before. The care of people with dementia has been radically affected by this new humanism. And yet, among all social issues, this is the one that is most deeply caught up in the contradictions, because the need is so intense and the size of the problem is so vast.

How matters will be resolved, in the long term, is impossible to know. There can be no doubt, however, that many profoundly positive changes have been taking place. Around 1980 the prevailing view of the conditions known as 'primary degenerative dementia' was that they presented a hopeless picture. Care for those who were affected was seen mainly as a matter of giving attention to basic physical needs while the process of degeneration in nerve tissue took its inexorable course. Generally it was believed that very little could be done in a truly therapeutic way through direct human intervention. No radical changes would be brought about until medical science had elucidated the underlying biochemistry and emerged with treatments that would arrest or prevent the pathological process. In effect, the *person* with dementia did not exist; 'going senile' was a sentence to radical exclusion.

Now, however, the whole situation looks very different. There is a growing awareness of how much can be done to enable people who have dementia to retain their well-being, and even many of their abilities, simply through better care practice and provision. At the same time we are coming to terms with the sobering fact that the achievements of biomedical research thus far have been very limited, despite a prodigious expenditure of effort, talent and financial resources. The biggest improvements in quality of life have not come from medical breakthroughs, but from the recognition of personhood in those who have dementia, and its many practical applications.

The emergence of the person in dementia care

The old culture of 'care' for those suffering from mental distress, formed and re-formed over 400 years ago or so, was deeply dehumanising, as many historical studies have shown (e.g. Foucault 1967; Ussher 1991). Dementia became a major feature in this scene only during the 20th century, as a result of the great demographic changes that created, on average, a much older population. Those who were put in the institutions tended to receive the very worst forms of care, and working in psychogeriatric settings was widely considered to bring little professional interest or personal reward. For many years, none of the main professions that were involved did anything strategic to improve the quality of care, and the personhood of those who had dementia was generally not considered.

The first real glimmer of hope came from the practice known as Reality Orientation. The origins of this lay in the rehabilitation of men who had been traumatised by war; it was an attempt to help restore them to the stability of civilian life. When Reality Orientation was taken into work with confused older people its good effects, in the form of renewed vitality and hopefulness, were clearly visible (Taulbee and Folsom 1966). Later research confirmed its beneficial effects, at least in some contexts (Holden and Woods 1995). It was all too easy, of course, to apply Reality Orientation in crude, crass and insensitive ways, and even to turn it into an instrument of oppression – an attempt to conform people to a 'reality' that was not their own. Nevertheless, Reality Orientation was the first sustained attempt to recognise the personhood of people with dementia, expressing the belief that they were not to be written off; it was worth taking the trouble to try to bring them back into a 'normal' way of life.

A few years after Reality Orientation had taken hold, another positive approach was developed, termed Validation Therapy (Feil 1982, 1993). Here there was a dramatic move away from the prevailing emphasis on cognition towards the realm of feelings and emotions, where dementia often brings far less impairment. This marked a big step forward in the care of people with dementia; above all it expressed a belief that their experience is to be taken with the utmost seriousness – and not dismissed, or 'corrected', as was so common in care practice. This humanitarian belief was taken even further in the approach known as Resolution Therapy, with its emphasis on developing empathy and communication (Stokes and Goudie 1989).

Another major contribution was the development of reminiscence work, along with the assimilation of biographical information into care practice (Gibson 1991, 1994). The crucial recognition here was that people with dementia, like the rest of us, are historical beings, whose identity is inextricably linked to their personal 'narrative'. The value of reminiscence lies partly in the sense of orientation and stability that it provides; it can be very reassuring – for some at least – to renew contact with the memories of people, places and activities from former times. As reminiscence work developed it became clear, too, that the past can provide metaphorical resources for people to talk about their present situation (Cheston 1996; Sutton 1995).

After the evident success of practices such as these, many ways of enriching the lives of people with dementia were explored: for example, music, dance, drama and graphic art (Jones and Miesen 1993, 1995). One of the most recent additions to this array is the use of various methods to provide pleasurable stimulation to the senses, bypassing cognition almost entirely (Benson 1994). Each of these forms of intervention, at its best, embodies a fuller recognition of those who have dementia as sentient beings, still capable of communicating their desires and feelings, and of living in a world of relationships. More details concerning these and other practices are to be found in Chapter 10 of this volume.

Around ten years ago it was virtually inconceivable that psychotherapy might be possible with people who have dementia. The common assumption was that they had no insight, and that, lacking the retentive power of memory, they would not be able to consolidate any of the changes that did take place (Kitwood 1990a). Now, however, several forms of therapeutic work are being explored: with individuals, with couples and with groups. In innovations such as these, a further dimension is added to the reinstatement of people with dementia; for the possibility is being considered that some form of 'personal growth' can occur, even in the face of cognitive decline.

In several countries there have been moves to design new patterns of group living, where people with dementia largely fend for themselves, but with a small background input of care. One of the best known of these is the Domus Project in Britain. Unlike some new schemes, this one has been evaluated, and the evidence is promising. There is a greater level of interaction, a decrease in depression and a lower rate of general decline, as compared with more traditional settings (Murphy, Lindesay and Dean 1994). New work is currently underway in sheltered housing, again suggesting that when attention is given to the meeting of psychological needs, this form of accommodation is far better suited to people with dementia than was previously believed (Petre 1995, 1996).

This is only a small fragment of the story of the transformation of attitudes and practices in dementia care. A detailed review, together with an appraisal of some of the relevant research, is given by Holden and Woods (1995). The cumulative weight of experience and systematic inquiry points overwhelmingly to two conclusions. The first is that people with dementia are far more resourceful, in virtually every aspect of life, than they were once assumed to be. They can learn new skills, if given sufficient time; they can give support to each other; they have much to tell us, if only we will listen – as Chapter 7 by Goldsmith makes clear. The second conclusion is that the course of a primary degenerative dementia is far less fixed than was formerly believed; it is open to change as a result of purely human intervention. Powerful evidence on this topic is to be found in the current series on person-centred care in the *Journal of Dementia Care* (see Kitwood 1995a). Surprisingly, however, in most of the positive initiatives to which I have referred above, very little attempt was made to give a systematic explication of the concept of personhood itself. Indeed, in some cases the theory that accompanied a particular form of practice was clearly inadequate. Reality Orientation, for example, was unjustified in seeing the person primarily as a cognitive being; Validation Therapy had a tendency to see problems overmuch as lying in the past rather than the present, and within the individual rather than in the social milieu (Kitwood 1994). From the period when care was beginning to improve there is, however, one statement that stands out above all others. This is the document, *Living Well into Old Age*, published by the King's Fund in 1986. Here it is plainly stated that people with dementia are individuals, and that they have the same value, the same needs and the same rights as everyone else. This was the first time – in Britain at least – that the ethical issues were clearly exposed, and that people with dementia were explicitly brought into the arena of moral concern.

The concept of personhood

It is vitally important to fill the theoretical void concerning personhood in dementia, if the many people committed to good practice are to gain in confidence and find a voice. The concept itself lies at the meeting point between two different kinds of discourse, the one ethical and the other social-psychological (Kitwood 1990b). Roughly speaking, the ethical discourse is concerned with what we ought to do, while the social-psychological discourse is concerned with how to do it. If we take this view, the term 'personhood' means a standing or status, bestowed on one individual by others; and there are empirical grounds for knowing whether or not personhood is being maintained. Some philosophers have tended to take the concept mainly as a component of moral theory (Quinton 1973). There are also theorists who have taken personhood simply as a psychological category. Tobin (1991), for example, makes it roughly equivalent to the idea of psychological resilience, in the face of much that might undermine a person in old age. However, it is when the concept of personhood retains both its ethical and its social-psychological meaning that it serves its proper function. At the heart of the ethic that underpins the concept of personhood lies the Kantian principle that each person should be treated as an end and never as a means to some other end (Mackie 1977). Kant attempted to provide a purely humanistic justification for this principle, taking rational argument to its outer limits; a similar doctrine, however, is to be found in the highest ethical teaching of each of the main religions and spiritual paths. The principle still leaves open the question of who is to be taken as a person, and on what basis. If autonomy and the fully developed use of reason are taken as criteria – as has often been the case in popular thinking – then people with dementia (like others with severe mental disabilities) are not worthy of inclusion. Here is the perfect rationalisation for 'uncare'. If, however, emotion, feeling and relational capability are taken as the key criteria, those who have dementia are undoubtedly to be viewed as persons. This view has recently been set out with great eloquence by Post (1995), who suggests an additional principle, that of moral solidarity: essentially that we should stand by people who have dementia, and never exclude them because of the failing of their mental powers.

At the social-psychological level, I would like to suggest that a model or theory of personhood suited to our purpose should meet the following criteria. First, it must be reflexive: that is, the categories that are used to describe or explain one group of people (in this case, those who have dementia) must be applicable in principle to the 'professionals' who use them (Little 1972). This is not only a methodological, but also a moral requirement. Second, it must view the person as a social being, not as a monad as has so often been the case in clinical work and in reductionistic theory (Burkitt 1993). That is why a moral theory that speaks of persons and obligations is more powerful than one which merely speaks of individuals and their 'rights'. Third, it must be developmental, showing how people can change – for good or ill – throughout the span of life. Fourth, it must bring out some of the most relevant psychological differences between people: doing what the blander forms of psychometric work simply cannot do (Harré 1976). Fifth, it must be compatible with what neuroscience tells us about how the brain develops and functions, both in health and in disease. Sixth, it must shed light on the psychological predicament of people who have dementia and suggest what they might need. Finally, it should be able to tell us something about the nature and meaning of good dementia care.

The psychology of personal being

It is a difficult and daunting task to create a model of the person which meets all seven criteria, and it can be done in several different ways. What follows here is no more than a sketch, building on some of my own earlier work (Kitwood 1987, 1989, 1990c, 1993, 1996). In effect, the model that I have developed brings together the frameworks of symbolic interactionism and depth psychology: the former dealing with the manifest aspects of social life, and the latter with processes that are said to be 'unconscious'.

The developmental study of infancy and childhood gives us a rich picture of the emergence of the psychological self, the sense of 'I'. There are many stages on the journey: the forming of attachments, the acquisition of a sense of agency (an ability to 'make things happen'), the realisation that many people exist in the world, the acceptance of experience that involves both pleasure and pain. One of the biggest steps is the acquisition of language, for when that is acquired there is not simply a self, but also a self-concept: a 'Me' as well as an 'I'.

There are vast differences in the quality of early relational experience, depending on the extent to which the key figures in a child's life are responsive, available, consistent and resourceful. It does not appear that perfection is required – simply a form of care-giving that is 'good enough' (Winnicott 1973). The tragedy is that for many children even this modest standard is not met; there is an excessive amount of privation and uncertainty, and in some cases outright cruelty and oppression. Whatever may be the case, each child, sooner or later, has to come to terms with a world that is often harsh, competitive and hypocritical, and to find a way of surviving within it. Here is the origin of what has been called the 'false self': formed not in joy, trust and creativity, but in adaption and survival. When virtually all of a child's development is around the false self there is an extreme of alienation and isolation, sometimes described as a schizoid state (Fairbairn 1952).

The idea of two types of 'self', two main patterns of development, runs right through those psychologies that are concerned with the promotion of personal 'growth' and positive change. In Jung's work it appears primarily as a distinction between ego and Self, but also as that between persona and shadow. The ego is formed through taking on some of the variety of roles that are provided, ready made, by society. On the basis of ego each person gives life a direction and finds a niche. Problems arise if living according to ego is too restrictive, if too much potential remains unexplored and undeveloped. According to Jung that is why some people have existential crises in mid-life; the prime task of later years is to move away from ego to develop a greater wholeness and completeness; this is the movement towards the Self (Jung 1933).

Parallels to these ideas are to be found in the work of several of the humanistic psychologists. For Rogers the issue was one of congruence: of there being a match between what a person is actually undergoing, what they are experiencing, and what they are presenting to others (Rogers 1961). In Transactional Analysis it comes in a more elaborated form, but the key issue is the distinction between the 'ego states' of the adapted child and the free child. The adapted child arises as a result of conformity to others' expectations, and particularly to pressures from critical or controlling parents; in some cases, too, from the attempt to avoid abuse or violence. The free child state, in contrast, expresses a condition where a person is able to be spontaneous, sensuous and intimate, and where the prime activity is play (Stewart and Joines 1987).

There are difficulties if the disjuncture is forced too far, and especially if a radical divide is posited between a false self and one which is somehow 'true', existing outside any real social context. (Whatever one might assume at a metaphysical level is a different matter). We can, however, legitimately use the terms 'adapted self' and 'experiential self'. The former refers to the person as highly and tightly socialised, particularly in relation to the performing of given roles. Sometimes, but not always, adaption involves both falsehood and estrangement. The experiential self, in contrast, arises from being with others in conditions of equality, mutual attention and mutual respect: what I have described elsewhere as 'moral space' (Kitwood 1990b). There is a famous distinction between two fundamentally different types of relationship: I–It and I–Thou (Buber 1922). Part, but by no means all, of the adapted self might be seen as a reaction to being treated as an 'it', an object. The experiential self is formed and nourished in the context of I–Thou relating.

We can use these ideas to explore some of the ways in which each person is unique. There are differences between individuals in their patterns of adaption, according to their social circumstances. Some of these patterns are relatively benign, especially where roles give scope for personal expression and moral commitment. This, however, is not always the case; some roles are degrading and dehumanising in themselves, and many kinds of stress arise from the different forms of role conflict. There are also great differences in the extent to which the experiential self develops. One key source of evidence here is the vast amount of reflection that has taken place on the experience of counselling and psychotherapy. Rogers (1961), for example, has described a continuum of 'personal growth'. At one end is a stage in which there is virtually no ability to experience or communicate on the feeling level, while at the other feelings are experienced in their richness and variety, are freely expressed and are used as a source of learning about the self. Furthermore, there are differences in the manner in which the experiential and adapted selves are related; the development of one does not necessarily imply the development of the other. An individual might, for example, have a highly elaborated 'front', or persona, and yet have an extraordinarily impoverished inner life.

At a very general level this model is applicable to all people, regardless of age, sex, class or society, although the categories which supply the content will vary from one culture to another. While the model is certainly one which professionals such as doctors, nurses and social workers can use in trying to understand their clients, it is also one which they can apply instructively to themselves. The model makes sense in neurological terms, if we accept the assumption of ontological monism: that there is only one (exceedingly complex) reality, which we attempt to describe in a number of different discourses. The brain is now recognised as a highly adaptive organ; interneuronal circuits are being continually formed and re-formed in response to the new learning that the organism requires (Damasio 1995). Each time that a new role is learned, for example, brain structures are established to enable the tasks to be performed efficiently; and when a role is ended these structures are slowly dismantled. Similarly, there is a neuronal counterpart to the experiential self; and as a person's experiential frame is enlarged, there are corresponding changes in brain structure. Presumably, also, those processes that are termed 'ego defence' (repression, denial, rationalisation, displacement etc.) are instantiated at a neurological level; in some cases through the deactivation of those proto-structures through which certain events or conflicts might have been consciously experienced.

We can use the model also to illustrate how each person develops through the life course. The adapted self is elaborated in many ways, but primarily through the taking on of new roles. Thus it proliferates throughout childhood and adolescence, with each step in the enlargement of skill, opportunity and social life. The process continues into adulthood, as a person enters the world of work (or unemployment), and perhaps takes on new responsibilities such as a committed relationship, parenting or the running of a home. With many people, it seems to be the case that the adapted self reaches its highest level of elaboration in the age period around 40–60, when roles and responsibilities are being added faster than they are being lost. Later life, for many people, brings a dismantling of the adapted self. Some major roles, such as that of parent or employee, are relinquished; a lowered income or problems of ill-health may cause a further diminution. The theorists of disengagement saw this as part of the natural progression of life. There is much evidence, however, to support a contrary view. Many people who make a success of their old age have managed to maintain a high level of engagement, perhaps taking on new but less demanding roles (Stevenson 1989).

The story of the experiential self is, to a large extent, that of the person in contexts of I–Thou relating, for it is here that it becomes possible to develop a subtle, sensitive and responsive way of being with others, and an 'inner discourse' of feeling and emotion (Hobson 1985). Where the experiential self does not develop well, this is in part a consequence of a person being subjected to oppression, conflict, rejection and exploitation – and, more rarely, actual trauma. The human organism is too sensitive to be able to bear these things in isolation, and so processes of defence exist to ward off an excess of anxiety or pain. The experiential self, however, is presented with many opportunities for development throughout life, particularly through love, friendship and spiritual commitment; a small minority find help through some form of therapy or counselling. There is no fundamental reason why the experiential self should not continue to grow in the later years and even, as clearly happens in some cases, during the course of a terminal illness. Much, however, in the process of ageing (as it has been constructed in contemporary industrial societies, at least), tends to hinder growth and to engender defensiveness, apathy or depression.

This model of personal being, which could be elaborated in much greater depth and detail, seems to meet the first five of the criteria which I suggested would be necessary for conceptualising personhood in the context of dementia care. It is reflexive, social and developmental; it reveals interpersonal differences; and it is compatible with neuroscientific knowledge. The last two criteria were that it should be directly relevant to the predicament of people who have dementia, and that it should be capable of shedding light on the meaning of good care. These are the two topics to which we shall now turn.

The agenda for dementia care

The concepts of experiential and adapted self can tell us much about the predicament of people who have dementia. Almost always, during the years before any cognitive deficits became noticeable, there have been losses in the adapted self. This can be illustrated by the example of two women from my psychobiographical research (Kitwood 1990c). For the first, the loss happened in several small stages; one bereavement succeeded another, and her life gradually closed in due to a decline in her general health. For the second, it happened through a single dramatic transition. She had spent almost all of her adult life in Southern Rhodesia, where she ran a hotel. When she returned to Britain, around the time of Independence, she lost her entire way of life, and found herself in what was virtually a foreign country. From a purely psychological point of view, both women were in a highly vulnerable position; their social connectedness, via the adapted self, had been greatly weakened. With the onset of dementia the adapted self almost always undergoes a further reduction, largely because of the inability or unwillingness of other people to support existing roles (Sabat and Harré 1992). If a person goes into residential care there is likely to be a further diminution. In the old-style institutional regimes many of the last vestiges of the adapted self were taken away and a single new role was created – that of inmate. If the inmate was also 'senile', virtually all was lost (Meacher 1972).

The experiential self, too, is imperilled through the process of dementia. There is a little evidence to suggest that people in whom it is only poorly developed may actually be at risk of developing dementia (for example, Oakley 1965). As cognitive impairment advances, the experiential frame is profoundly disturbed. Failures of memory and judgement are alarming in themselves, but they may also bring secondary consequences such as delusions (essentially a misattribution of causes). Desperate needs for comfort and security come to the surface. Those who remain walled off by defences are protected for a while, but when the defences eventually break down there may be a powerful invasion of emotion which they have no capacity to understand. A small proportion of people also have to endure hallucinations, and here their isolation is profound.

The aim of dementia care, in the broadest sense, is to maintain personhood in the face of advancing cognitive impairment. Through the concepts of experiential self and adapted self it is possible to see what this means in a little more detail. The principles that underlie the points that follow apply across all contexts of care, because they relate primarily to the existential plight of the person with dementia. However, some of the realities are more complex and difficult when care-giving has taken over from a relationship of another, and more mutual, kind; for here both parties have already made deep psychological investments.

Taking care of the adapted self means, essentially, enabling a person to continue, as far as possible and for as long as possible, in familiar roles. Each role provides, so to speak, a 'beaten track', where a way of being and doing has been deeply learned. Each role, also, is an arena where a person is recognised, acknowledged and integrated into a form of life that is shared with others. When a person with dementia is living at home it is possible for some roles, such as grandparent, host, shopper and gardener, to continue to some degree. Imaginative help may be needed to provide parts of the action that a person cannot now carry out alone; and in some instances the problems lie with the sequencing, not with the actions themselves. As cognitive impairment advances it is inevitable that some roles will have to be relinquished (driver or domestic accountant, for example), and here it is vital to help the person with dementia to maintain a sense of self-worth and significance in the face of loss. Very similar issues arise in the contexts of formal care, where people with dementia often want to contribute something, rather then just be passive receivers. It is not uncommon, for example, for a person to frame attendance at a day centre as 'going to work', and in some cases at least, there is work that they can do, particularly in helping to care for others. All too often the needs of the adapted self have been ignored, perhaps because care-givers are too insistent on their own projects or too committed to order and control.

The more joyous and fulfilling aspects of dementia care, however, both for receiver and giver, are likely to be on the basis of the experiential self. The central point here is that a person with dementia still has an emotional and relational life, even though without the stabilisation and compensation that cognitions ordinarily provide. One kind of interaction in dementia care is 'holding': providing a safe space where it is possible to experience psychological pain without being overwhelmed. A person might, for example, be subject to terrifying hallucinations, but these are just bearable if he or she is in actual physical contact with a carer who is known and trusted. Another type of interaction is validation; not in the sense of a total 'therapy', but simply acknowledging the subjective truth of a person's experience, without an obsessional concern with 'cognitive rectification'. Yet another type of interaction might be termed 'timulation': a neologism which means providing pleasurable stimulation to the senses, but in a way that respects a person's boundaries and values. Here there is the opportunity for simple sensuous enjoyment without the demands of thought or the restrictions imposed by a harsh and critical moralism. A further example is 'celebration': simply sharing in the beauty, the fun and the joy of living, where the free child is welcomed and encouraged. Strikingly, it is often in episodes of celebration, such as parties, outings and dances, that people who have dementia behave most 'normally', and the us–them barriers dissolve away to nothing.

As yet we do not know the full range of possibilities for the experiential self, when the care is of a very supportive and empowering kind. The first glimpses are now appearing of a different long-term pattern of dementia, in which people do not inevitably decline into vegetation. Some, at least, may actually be enabled to undergo a form of personal growth which even surprises and delights their relatives: becoming less obsessive, more trustful, or emerging from depression into a state of acceptance and tranquillity (Kitwood 1995b). The overall pattern cannot be described at present; that will only be possible after a large body of evidence has been collected.

Finally, this brief exploration of personhood gives us small glimpses of the skills and sensitivities that are required in those who are involved in care-giving. A good careworker must, of course, be thoroughly competent in all the standard tasks which the job entails, and in that sense be well adapted to the role; the same applies, although in a less formal sense, to a family member or a friend who has become a carer. But beyond that, effective care-giving requires a well-developed experiential self. This involves being familiar with the world of feeling and emotion; being willing to bear the burden that arises from attachment; being comfortable with an intimacy that needs no words; and being capable of play. In counselling and psychotherapy the central quality required of a practitioner is sometimes described as that of giving 'free attention'. This is not learned as mere technique, but arises through real development. A person becomes more insightful and self-accepting, less distracted by inner conflict and anxiety; and hence more able to set his or her own issues on one side for the sake of another. A similar quality is needed, and to a high degree, in dementia care. One encouraging sign is that some family carers are able to move in this direction if they are well supported, even while they are enduring so much suffering and stress (Coates 1995).

Looking to the future

There can be no doubt about the tremendous progress that has been made in recent years, as a new culture of dementia care has gradually come into being. Each chapter of this book demonstrates this in some way. If good care, in all its aspects, is seen as a kind of mosaic, it seems likely that many of the individual pieces have already been found (Kitwood 1995a). One of the tasks that lies ahead is fitting them all together to create the whole rich pattern, and here a clear conception of personhood is essential. Beyond that, there is the problem of actually setting up the services that embody what we know, with all the training and personal development which that implies. This is a difficult and daunting task, not least because there are so many countervailing forces: negative traditions in care practice, the severe lack of public funding, and the many corrupting pressures of the market. There is also a huge research task in investigating the consequences of new practices and, in contrast to much biomedical work, this holds the promise of immediate benefits.

Among the historically new features of our time, none is more significant than the widespread presence of people with dementia. If we fail them at this point, it will not be because of a lack of knowledge, but because our social, educational, political and economic arrangements are inadequate to the task. If we succeed, it will be one of the most hopeful signs that it is yet possible to build a society in which compassion and integrity prevail.

References

Benson, S. (1994) 'Sniff and doze therapy.' *Journal of Dementia Care 2*, 1, 11–15.

Buber, M. (1922) *I and Thou*. English translation by Ronald Gregor Smith (1937). Edinburgh: Clark.

Burkitt, I. (1993) *Social Selves*. London: Sage.

Cheston, R. (1996) 'Stories and metaphors: talking about the past in a psychotherapy group for persons with dementia.' *Ageing and Society 16*, 579–602.

Coates, D. (1995) 'The process of learning in dementia–carer support programmes: some preliminary observations.' *Journal of Advanced Nursing 21*, 41–46.

Damasio, A.R. (1995) *Descartes' Error*. London: Picador.

Fairbairn, W.R.D. (1952) *Psychoanalytic Studies of the Family*. London: Routledge and Kegan Paul. (See, especially, Chapter 1).

Feil, N. (1982) *Validation: the Feil Method*. Cleveland: Edward Feil Productions.

Feil, N. (1993) *The Validation Breakthrough*. Baltimore: Health Promotions Press.

Foucault, M. (1967) *Madness and Civilization*. London: Tavistock.

Gibson, F. (1991) *A Positive Approach to Dementia*. Jordanstown: University of Ulster.

Gibson, F. (1994) *Reminiscence and Recall*. London: Ace Books.

Harré, R. (ed) (1976) *Personality.* Oxford: Blackwell.

Hobson, R.E. (1985) *Forms of Feeling.* London: Tavistock.

Holden, U. and Woods, R. (1995) *Positive Approaches to Dementia Care.* Edinburgh: Churchill Livingstone.

Jones, G.M.M. and Miesen, B.M.L. (1993) *Caregiving in Dementia.* London: Routledge.

Jones, G.M.M. and Miesen, B.M.L. (eds) (1995) *Caregiving in Dementia.* Volume II. London: Routledge.

Jung, C.G. (1993) *Modern Man in Search of Soul.* London: Routledge and Kegan Paul. (See, especially, Chapter 5.)

King's Fund (1986) *Living Well into Old Age: Applying Principles of Good Practice to Services for Elderly People with Severe Mental Impairments.* London: The King's Fund.

Kitwood, T.M. (1987) 'Dementia and its pathology: in brain, mind or society?' *Free Associations 8,* 81–93.

Kitwood, T.M. (1989) 'Brain, mind and dementia: with particular reference to Alzheimer's disease.' *Ageing and Society 9,* 1–15.

Kitwood, T.M. (1990a) 'Psychotherapy and dementia.' *Psychotherapy Section Newsletter 8,* 40–56.

Kitwood, T.M. (1990b) *Concern for Others.* London: Methuen.

Kitwood, T.M. (1990c) 'Understanding senile dementia: a psychobiographical approach.' *Free Associations 19,* 60–76.

Kitwood, T.M. (1993) 'Towards a theory of dementia care: the interpersonal process.' *Ageing and Society 13,* 15–67.

Kitwood, T.M. (1994) 'Review of *The Validation Breakthrough* (by Naomi Feil).' *Journal of Dementia Care 2,* 6, 29–30.

Kitwood, T.M. (1995a) 'Building up the mosaic of good practice: introducing a new series in person-centred care.' *Journal of Dementia Care 3,* 5, 12–13.

Kitwood, T.M. (1995b) 'Positive long term changes in dementia: some preliminary observations.' *Journal of Mental Health 4,* 133–144.

Kitwood, T.M. (1996) 'The concept of personhood and its implications for the care of those who have dementia.' In G.M.M. Jones and B.M.L. Miesen (eds) *Caregiving in Dementia.* Volume II. London: Routledge.

Little, B.R. (1972) 'Psychological man as humanist scientist and specialist.' *Journal of Experimental Research in Psychiatry 6,* 95–118.

Mackie, J.L. (1977) *Ethics.* Harmondsworth: Penguin.

Meacher, M. (1972) *Taken for a Ride.* London: Longmans.

Murphy, E., Lindesay, J. and Dean, M. (1994) *The Domus Project.* London: The Sainsbury Centre.

Oakley, D.P. (1965) 'Senile dementia – some aetiological factors.' *British Journal of Psychiatry 111,* 414–419.

Petre, T. (1995) 'Dementia and sheltered housing.' In T. Kitwood, S. Buckland and T. Petre (eds) *Brighter Futures: A Report on Research into Provision for Persons with Dementia in Residential Homes, Nursing Homes and Sheltered Housing.* Anchor Housing Association (in collaboration with Methodist Homes for the Aged).

Petre, T. (1996) 'Back into the swing of her sociable life.' *Journal of Dementia Care 4, 1,* 24–25.

Post, S. (1995) *The Moral Challenge of Alzheimer's Disease.* Baltimore: Johns Hopkins Press.

Quinton, A. (1973) *The Nature of Things.* London: Routledge.

Rogers, C.R. (1961) *On Becoming a Person.* Boston: Houghton Mifflin.

Sabat, S. and Harré, R. (1992) 'The construction and deconstruction of self in Alzheimer's disease.' *Ageing and Society 12,* 443–461.

Stevenson, O. (1989) *Age and Vulnerability.* London: Edward Arnold.

Stewart, I and Joines, V. (1987) *TA Today.* Nottingham: Lifespace Publications.

Stokes, G. and Goudie, F. (1989) *Working With Dementia.* Bicester: Winslow.

Sutton, L. (1995) *Whose memory is it anyway?* Unpublished PhD thesis, University of Southampton.

Taulbee, L.R. and Folsom, J.C. (1966) 'Reality orientation for geriatric patients.' *Hospital and Community Psychiatry 17,* 133–135.

Tobin, S.S. (1991) *Personhood in Advanced Old Age.* New York: Springer.

Ussher, J.M. (1991) *Women's Madness: Misogyny or Mental Illness?* London: Harvester.

Winnicott, D.W. (1973) *The Child, The Family and the Outside World.* Harmondsworth: Penguin.

Chapter 2

Ethical Dilemmas in Care and Research for People with Dementia

Alan Jacques

The ethical issues which arise during the course of a long and complicated disorder such as dementia are many and various. Here I hope to give an overview of some of these issues from a personal vantage point. My own experience is, first, as an old age psychiatrist in a multidisciplinary team with strong community links, working in an area with an effective social work (social services) department and a thriving voluntary sector; second, as a member of Scotland's Alzheimer's interest groups, now united in Alzheimer Scotland – Action on Dementia, which have taken particular interest in law reform within Scotland's separate legal system; and third, as a member of our national 'watch-dog' body for the welfare of people with mental disorders, including dementia. I hope this experience brings together practical issues, a local perspective and general principles. Many of the issues relate to decision-making.

Decision-making in dementia

During the 10 to 15 years of dementia, as the person moves from his or her normal self to terminal incapacity, there is a huge number of day-to-day and major decisions which need to be made (Table 2.1), and there tends to be different ground rules and legal provisions in each of these areas. Day-to-day decisions, about whether to wash, what to wear, eat or engage in, who to mix with, etc. are not covered by law, but it is often the case that if these decisions are not made, or inadvisedly made, one or other of the major decisions may have to follow. Financial and health care decisions may be big or small to professionals but all are likely to be important to the individual. Welfare decisions usually relate to the acceptance of intervention or care at home, attendance at day centres, or residential respite or long-term care. Decisions

Table 2.1 Decision-making in dementia (1)

Day-to-day
Financial
  Management of affairs
  Wills
Welfare
Health Care
  Physical
  Mental (dementia and its psychiatric complications)
Research
  Treatment of dementia
  Non-treatment
  Non-dementia

about dementia itself may include questions of genetic testing, early diagnosis, treatments to slow the progress of the illness, assessment and management of behaviour disturbance, and terminal care. Research decisions are becoming more and more relevant as money is poured into the effort to understand the nature of the illnesses causing dementia, to find treatments, and to understand and treat symptoms.

In all these decisions the person may choose a course of action, or have given prior or proxy indication of choice, may reject a choice, may vary in which way to turn, may fail to choose, or may have a choice and fail to communicate it. Choices may be deemed invalid. Based on this, or on failure to choose, the law provides in some cases for a court-appointed agent to make decisions on the person's behalf.

How do people with dementia fare with all these decisions? In order to reach a decision on any particular problem we must recognise that there is a problem and form an opinion of what the problem is. We have to keep it in mind for long enough to reach a decision. We need to be able to formulate on some level a solution or choice of solutions. We are likely to want to have some ideas on the risks and benefits of accepting or rejecting possible solutions, or, just as important, of not coming to a decision. If others are involved in our chosen solution we must be able to communicate with them, sometimes in quite a formal way. In coming to our decision we may be influenced to a greater or lesser extent by other people. We may even allow them to make the decision for us. But it remains our choice that we do so. We have a general right (which

Table 2.2 Decision-making in dementia (2)

Failing abilities
Perception
Understanding
Connections and logical thinking
Memory
Motivation
Dysphasia and dysgraphia
Loss of control
Standards
Planning
Judgement
Conscience and moral sense
Reaction to the experience of dementia
Anxiety, depression
Dependence on others
Suspicion
Denial

may be limited by laws) to make choices which others might consider unwise or wrong.

In all these stages of decision-making the person suffering dementia is potentially in difficulties right from the beginning of the illness, and will be in gradually increasing difficulties as it progresses (Table 2.2). Take the decision which 'should' follow if, say, a lady with dementia is failing to cook adequately and repeatedly burning pots. This failure is a clear change from her previous normal self (an important point – in all assessments related to a person's competence we must be careful to make a comparison with that person's pre-morbid abilities, attitudes, style etc., not with some statistical or social norm: commonly used rating scales and other assessment tools frequently fail to recognise this point). If the failure was due to physical disability we might expect the lady to organise simpler cooking arrangements, use carry-in meals, ask for a home help, or even decide to give up living alone; there are many possible choices. Personality, past experience, social networks, future plans, current mood state, the influences of family, friends and professionals and other factors will determine the preferred solution.

Loss of the ability to perceive

The person with dementia may not perceive what is happening, even if she can see those burnt pots perfectly well. She may not recognise these are her particular pots burning. She may especially have difficulty in understanding the implications and risk of burning pots – the more abstract aspects of the problem. She may not understand the warnings given by others. She is likely, even in the early stages of dementia, to forget the episodes quickly, or not retain the information long enough to collect it all together so as to decide what to do.

Damage to connections within the brain is a fundamental feature of all forms of dementia, so it is not surprising that sufferers have difficulty with connecting this perception with that, thinking through problems in any sort of logical fashion, or relating a perceived problem with potential solutions. In addition, the abstract thinking required to consider these various options and look at their risks and benefits is equally likely to be impaired from quite early on in dementia.

Similarly, the output of the brain, the direction of our speech and behaviour, and particularly the more sophisticated, highly co-ordinated aspects, are impaired in dementia. Our lady may recognise the problem posed and reach conclusions about what should be done, but she may be unable to co-ordinate the necessary actions to deal with the risks to her and her neighbours. Or she may have difficulty in communicating her decision coherently. Moreover, her ability to feel and express emotion, her drive and motivation are likely to be diminished as well. She may grasp the problem, work out its solution, see the risks of doing nothing, but simply not be bothered to do anything about it – an immensely frustrating experience for her carers.

Loss of the ability to monitor

These impairments of ability are the core of dementia. In addition there is a vast range of brain functions involving the monitoring of all our activities. Most of this monitoring is unconscious, some is conscious. Before any action we have intentions, based on some sort of aim or standard. During the action we monitor how we are fitting in with our standard or plan. Afterwards we judge whether we have achieved our aim, met our standards, done right or wrong. So the lady burning pots may have had difficulties in planning how to cook her meal safely, may not monitor safety as carefully as usual during the cooking and may not have judged her performance accurately afterwards. What is more, this monitoring and comparison with performance or moral standards will also come into the decision-making process. If the lady cannot set her standards and monitor them for cooking a pot of soup, how can she be expected to set standards and monitor her decisions: 'Is it right for me to have a home help?', 'How do I go about it properly?', 'Was that the right decision?'.

The result of this decline in standard-setting and monitoring is likely to be that the person may make misguided decisions, or may be excessively vulnerable to the influence of others, even if that influence is malign. Again we are here describing a change from the person's normal self. We all know people without dementia who are undiscerning, illogical, incompetent or unwise. Only if there is a change have we any right to implicate dementia as the cause.

Reactions to the experience of dementia

The changes described so far are based on organic changes in the brain. On top of these, the reactions of sufferers to dementia are of great importance. If they experience, with insight, full or partial, the decline, problems, mistakes and risks of dementia, they may become anxious, over-cautious and too ready to hand over control of decisions to others. Or they may become depressed and indecisive. 'You tell me what to do, dear'. If, on the other hand, through lack of insight or denial, they experience a diverse crowd of busybodies advising or telling them to accept help they think they don't need, they are likely to be angry and reject the help on offer.

So, although dementia is a gradual process, decision-making on small and big issues is likely to be difficult. The sufferer's capacity to decide must always be in doubt. Incidentally, it is interesting to note, in relation to the assessment of capacity, that although it is relatively easy to test impairments in memory and other mental abilities reliably, it is at present extremely difficult to make an objective and accurate assessment of a person's monitoring processes and their vulnerability to outside influences – all the important areas of judgement and standards, moral sense etc. which are so important as a basis for sound decision-making.

Paternalism and best interests

On the basis of the many and complex organic mental changes and the reactive psychological changes that come with dementia we could readily come to the conclusion that, from the early stages onwards, sufferers are mentally incapable and that we, in our various caring roles, need to take over. We fill the gaps in their brain power by using ours for them, in their best interests and with an authority based on our role – the duty of family members to each other, the professionals' duty to care and not to neglect those in their charge. Family carers

Table 2.3 Paternalism

Patient	– infantilising
Carer	– implies goodwill, knowledge and commitment
Carers	– assumes agreement
The Law	– limited legal basis

regularly take decisions in this way, and professionals, particularly doctors and nurses (but not only they) have a long history of doing so.

This 'paternalism' (an interesting linking of male gender and parenthood to substitute decision-making) and its associated assumption of incapacity is tempting (Table 2.3). But it is becoming gradually less tenable. The well-meaning daughter who becomes a sort of 'mother' to her own dementing mother may believe she acts in good faith, but brings to the role all sorts of memories, attitudes and prejudices from their earlier relationship. She effectively infantilises her mother. Many, though by no means all, people with dementia do not like this. They feel that they are adults and do not like being treated like children. What is more, they are not like children. A child, even a mentally impaired child, has an organised developing brain. The person with dementia did have such a coherently functioning brain but its functions are now deteriorating in a *random* fashion. This degeneration is not orderly and cannot be considered the opposite of development.

Paternalism may work for the best interests of the person if we can assume that the carer has thorough knowledge of the person, goodwill towards him or her, and a commitment to being helpful and carrying their plans through. If these are absent, or if carers act for their own personal, professional or institutional interests, there are grave dangers of exploitation, abuse or neglect.

Paternalism would appear to assume that there is only one carer with one view. It does not help where there is a 'paternity' dispute between different carers' views. The most powerful carer is in danger of bullying the rest and dictating the decision.

Despite these dangers informal paternalism has worked well, when, for example, a well-intentioned caring family helps to organise finances on behalf of the sufferer, or introduces care services behind the sufferer's back but in their best interests and successfully. Carers' groups and Alzheimer's societies need to remind themselves frequently that they are mostly made up of such well-intentioned, altruistic, committed carers. There are also, however, uninterested, self-interested, malicious and split families. Some sufferers have no immediate family at all. They rely on the goodwill of professionals who have the complex task of acting paternalistically whilst protecting their charges' autonomy. These professionals are essentially strangers with no necessary personal commitment to the person with dementia. Good professional training, good knowledge of the client and respect for the person may make such professional paternalism work well. The 'best interests' of the person are seen to include an altruistic respect for how their wishes can be accommodated in the final decision.

Over the past 20 or 30 years there has been a gradual move within the hospital, public sector residential care and community care sectors, to see paternalism as a potential abuse of professional power. It is a fascinating reflection on the effects of deregulation, less hierarchical or bureaucratic structures, smaller units and the other features of some parts of the private care home sector and more isolated parts of the public sector, that paternalism survives strongly in a few places. While many care providers open their doors, remove physical restraints, avoid where possible drugs as a form of restraint and encourage personal autonomy, a few lock their doors, develop potentially intrusive surveillance systems, administer crushed-up tranquilliser tablets in the soup and make financial decisions behind the backs of dementing residents. But in all forms of care we need to ask how much we are to trust the automatic beneficence and wisdom of a nightshift care worker in a hospital or residential home, or an isolated sitter/carer in the person's home, if neither has regular supervision.

Autonomy or self-determination

If there are dangers in relying on paternalism, what of autonomy (Table 2.4)? There has been a world-wide trend to search for and find capacity for autonomy in all types of people with handicaps. Why should people with dementia not be seen in exactly the same way as people with paraplegia or deafness? The organic losses of function I described above, however, amount to a diminution of the person's personality, those memories which give them continuity, their very sense of identity. Their ability to understand, reason and respond is diminished. The person with dementia is, quite literally, less of a person than they were. Allowing free rein to paternalism to people in such circumstances is dangerous. But trying to encourage autonomy in people who are actually mentally incompetent is equally dangerous.

The person with dementia, not realising that there is a problem, or impaired in their ability to think rationally, may fail to make a necessary decision, or,

Table 2.4 Autonomy

Patient	Respects rights Ignores or plays down impairment May lead to neglect May leave person open to abuse

lacking judgement, may make a totally unwise one, or even come to a 'right' decision completely by accident.

There is a view, popular among some professionals, that the loss of judgement and inhibitions in dementia allows the person to do those rebellious things they never dared to do before ('when I am old I will wear purple'). This view is based on a misunderstanding of the nature of disinhibition in dementia. People with dementia lose self-control mechanisms in the brain, not by design but as a symptom of a dreadful illness, and in random fashion. Carers who encourage the view that dementia sufferers are in a second adolescent rebellion may possibly be themselves rebelling by proxy.

In assessing a person's ability to act autonomously in dementia, we need again to remind ourselves that we are comparing the person with their own norm. Some people never in their lives acted very autonomously – they relied on other people's advice far too much or repeatedly failed to make decisions. We cannot expect such people to become independent-minded and decisive in the middle of dementia. Reliance on the autonomy of the individual with dementia is tempting and politically correct, but does not fit well with an understanding of the nature and effects of dementia or of the people who suffer from it.

Legal provisions

Laws have been brought into use (or rather drifted into use) where paternalism and 'best interests' arguments are clearly dangerous and autonomy impossible (Table 2.5). The classic case is the relatively well-off person whose relatives cannot necessarily be trusted to act in the person's interest and have no legal right to act on his or her behalf, and where the person cannot say what or how his or her affairs are to be managed or suggests a manifestly unrealistic method of management. In Scotland a court can appoint an agent, called a Curator Bonis, to manage the affairs. This curatorship role is monitored by an official of the court. This and the Scottish laws relating to other decisions in dementia

Table 2.5 Scottish legal provisions

Finances
    Mandates and Social Security appointees
    Power of Attorney – appointed by the individual when competent
    Curator Bonis – court-appointed
    Hospital patient's finances – management by hospital managers
Welfare
    Mental Health Act Guardianship
    National Assistance Act
Health Care
    Physical – None
    Mental – Mental Health Act admission
Research
    None
Tutor Dative
    Welfare and physical health
Tutor-at-law
    All decisions

are imperfect, old-fashioned and usually derived originally for other purposes. The same is true in many other countries, though some have achieved law reform. In Scotland the Mental Health Act (which deals with admission to hospital for treatment or nursing care and guardianship for welfare) was devised for people with schizophrenia and other so-called functional mental illnesses (where the disorder of function seems out of proportion or unaccompanied by any organic changes) and for mental handicap. The financial provisions – power of attorney, granted by the individual when competent and Curator Bonis, appointed by a court are old common law appointments (that is, there are no statutes approved by parliament covering the appointments), with monitoring which is non-existent in the first instance and too intrusive and expensive in the second, except for those who can afford to pay. There is no statute law and almost no case law covering physical health care decisions. Research has hardly begun to be considered as a subject of legal interest in Scotland.

The legal provisions that we have are all-or-none – the person is deemed either competent or incompetent. This does not fit at all well with the gradually progressive nature of most dementias. Furthermore, the provisions that exist are split into the different functional areas listed in Table 2.1. A Curator Bonis can only act in relation to the person's financial affairs, not make welfare, health or research decisions; a mental health guardian has no financial authority. To ensure more wide-ranging powers solicitors have gone back to the 16th century and revived the position of 'Tutor Dative' – a court appointee who can make both welfare and physical health care decisions – and that of 'Tutor-at-Law' – the nearest male relative, appointed by a court to make all decisions for the person. These appointments are effectively unmonitored. The legal position has become ludicrous. Our outdated, clumsy and inappropriate laws cover only some of the possible decision-making problems of dementia and cover those unsatisfactorily.

Over the past ten years voluntary organisations dedicated to improving dementia care in Scotland have campaigned for law reform. Now the Scottish Law Commission, the job of which is to advise the government on possible legal changes, has provided a wide-ranging discussion document which, following two major consultation exercises, has led to final proposals and a draft bill. The new proposals, summarised briefly in Table 2.6, would bring simple ways of allowing family carers (and possibly some professional providers of care) to manage the day-to-day finances of incapable dementia sufferers. Powers of attorney would be better devised and monitored. It would be possible to appoint a welfare attorney, as well as a financial attorney. Advance health care directives, in the form of advance refusals of treatment (not including treatment covered by the Mental Health Act) would have legal binding except in certain circumstances. Court-appointed financial guardianship would be possible for people who do not have a lot of money. The powers of both financial and welfare guardians could vary from case to case, depending on the degree of incapacity of the person, thus allowing a degree of flexibility absent in the present all-or-none system. In addition to welfare guardianship, the court could authorise welfare interventions not needing a longer-term appointment. All these arrangements would be monitored in a variety of ways by an Office of 'Public Guardian' for financial matters and the Mental Welfare Commission for Scotland for matters of health and welfare. In addition there have been proposals for 'vulnerable adults' legislation which would allow access for assessment and intervention in cases of possible neglect or abuse.

It has seemed as if things are moving forwards and that gaps in the legal support for dementia sufferers and their carers would be filled in ways which would reflect the particular problems of dementia. However, the debates about new laws have raised some important questions. If informal arrangements have generally worked should we not trust to family duties, loyalties and privacy

Table 2.6 Law reform: Scottish proposals

Simple methods of financial management
Improved rules for powers of attorney
Welfare attorneys
Advance refusals for physical health care
Guardians with flexible powers for welfare and finances
Intervention orders
Monitoring by public guardian (finances) and mental welfare
    commission (welfare and health)
No proposals on research
Abuse – assessment and interventions

rather than have intensive and expensive laws (what might be called the 'family values' argument)? These laws could be seen as interfering with the liberty of individuals, particularly the liberty to make the 'wrong' decision (the 'civil liberties' argument).

How far should the law intrude into the already complicated lives of dementia sufferers and their families? On the one hand it is very easy to say that the sufferer is likely to be impaired in their capacity to make decisions. No one has the right, unless there is an appropriate legal provision, to make decisions for another adult. The law, it could be argued, should step in for all types of decision-making, not just be available to cover the finances of rich people and a few extreme cases. Scotland's population of 5,000,000 people includes maybe 60,000 individuals with significant degrees of dementia, often affecting their capacity to decide. All these people need protection.

Providing comprehensive protection would, however, be very costly. It would be time-consuming for families and professionals. It could actually inhibit carers from making perfectly reasonable 'best interests' decisions informally and so greatly complicate care decisions. It could create confusion for the sufferer, who would be faced with a bewildering array of agents, guardians and monitoring agencies on top of the already bewildering array of assessors and helpers. At the end of the day, there is no guarantee that legal interventions will bring 'better' decisions than informal arrangements in most cases. After all, in the present system there are, admittedly in a minority of instances, attorneys, curators, guardians or hospitals who have not acted in the best interests of the person with dementia.

Table 2.7 Implied or pseudo-autonomy

1. Staff Imposed	'They all like soup'
2. Relatives etc.	'She likes soup'
3. Prior Preferences	'She used to like soup'
4. Advocates	'I believe she likes soup'
5. Behavioural Consent	Soup eaten
6. Passive Acceptance	Allows feeding
7. Validation	'I like this hotel'
8. False Choice	'Yes' 'No'
9. Variable Choice	'Yes' 'No'

Implied autonomy

The drive to elevate self-determination as the highest principle, and the current gaps in legal provision have encouraged carers, both formal and informal, to search for evidence of autonomy, and sometimes we feel we have found it in forms which might be described as 'implied' or 'pseudo-autonomy' (Table 2.7). If we take a very simple example – the decision whether or not to take soup at lunchtime in a care home. The resident is not capable of deciding, or cannot communicate, or even seems to be refusing the soup. Staff are not clear what her real view is. First staff may assume that she would go along with their paternalistic views – they know what is good for her, in her best interests and that is to take the soup. It is simply assumed that she would agree if she could. This style is generally seen as old-fashioned and patronising. However, it can still be found, particularly among the enthusiasts for various dementia 'therapies'. Who said that every or even most dementia sufferers would wish to be involved in reality orientation, reminiscence, exercises, validation, music therapy, pet-assisted therapy, aromatherapy, spiritual exercises or single rooms? The enthusiasts did. The polite smile of a sufferer may easily be misread as positive acceptance of the theory behind these activities.

Second, we may rely on reports of previous preferences from relatives' accounts or from the sufferer. These and the more explicit advance directives are likely to lead to the most reliable guesses of present preferences. If she always liked soup or said, 'always remember to give me my soup' we feel reasonably safe to give it without her current consent. But there are some difficulties in relying too much on prior preferences (Table 2.8). The person's actual experience of dementia may differ quite dramatically from what she expected before it. Her preferences may actually change because of the dementia. There may be doubts about the validity of preferences if they were stated a long time ago, if they were made after the dementia began, if they were based on hearsay or if they seem eccentric.

The new world of advocacy has brought other attempts to interpret the person's prior or present views or best interests. But advocates are also 'guessing'. To be recognised as an authentic voice of the sufferer the advocate must base his or her guesses on a thorough knowledge of the person's past, of dementia and its effects on this individual, of the views of those with an interest in the person, of the choices available, and of risks and benefits from the various choices. They need to avoid bringing their own likes and dislikes or their own prejudices into the picture. It must be doubted if many such dispassionate and disinterested experts exist! So much of all our thinking about the experience of dementia is a reflection of our own views of what it must be like, of how we think we will react and our objective view of sufferers we have known. We need constantly to remind ourselves that it is almost impossible to understand the real experience of dementia, particularly in its later stages.

Table 2.8 Advance directives

1. **Reading the future**
   Experience of dementia – may not be as expected
   Effects of dementia –   wishes may change
   Therapeutic advances –   may change the possibilities
2. **Time**
   Duration of dementia –   any directive will be 'old' in late dementia
   Time of signing –   may reflect a different phase of life
3. **Incapacity**
   When does it occur –   when should directive take effect?
   Who decides –   the doctor, or should others be involved?
4. **Validity**
   Does it represent the person's normal wishes?
   Eccentric directives

We may look for clues about the person's preferences in her current muddled utterances or behaviour. She may allow staff to feed her without evidence of protest. This must have some validity, but if it were signing a large cheque rather than lifting a spoon we might be less certain. Currently fashionable 'validation' techniques even suggest that we can translate muddled or delusional statements into valid voices. This is possible also, but again relies greatly on the subjective interpretations of the therapist.

These pseudo-autonomies may assist in day-to-day decisions, but must surely be treated sceptically if used to justify major decisions, such as consent for operation or research or the decision to move to a care home. All such guesswork is subjective and not easily validated.

Unfortunately even apparently clear statements have to be doubted sometimes. The person may give or withhold consent quite unambiguously – we take this on face value but the decision has not been reached in a logical way or may be based on a misunderstanding of the problem. A person with dementia may retain the ability to read and write, even to understand individual words, but not understand the general implications of a sentence or a document, say a power of attorney. Families and professionals have been all too ready to accept the meaningless 'yes' and also to ignore the meaningless 'no'. Even worse is the position of the sufferer who repeatedly changes from definite 'yes' to definite 'no'.

Good practice guidelines

In the present legal system with its many gaps, and with the risks of allowing free rein to paternalism, autonomy or pseudo-autonomy, there have been some moves to regularise, by guidelines, what can be seen as good practice (Table 2.9). Even if new laws were to come in we should not expect all eventualities to be covered. There will always be a place for informal arrangements. We may not trust the person or their carers to make decisions that are necessary in the true best interests of all concerned and with fairness. But the law cannot afford to take over every decision.

In Scotland there is active debate on good practice guidelines on issues of restraint, consent for investigation, operation and medical treatment, intervention in cases of abuse or neglect, and management of finances for incapable people in community care (at present a total 'black hole' in legal provision, leaving people discharged from hospital with their funds permanently frozen). In all these areas guidelines emphasise proper assessment, particularly of risks, multidisciplinary and multi-agency involvement in place of isolated decision-

Table 2.9 Good practice guidelines

Restraint	Direct physical
	Mechanical
	Locked doors
	Surveillance
	Passive alarms
	Drugs
Health Care	Investigation
	Operation
	Medical and dental treatment etc.
Abuse	Physical
	Sexual
	Neglect
Finances	Incapable adults in Community Care

making, consensus, continuing monitoring of the case, the principle of minimum necessary intervention with reference to the person's present and prior expressed wishes, and the need actively to involve the sufferer as far as possible in all stages of the process.

Where are we just now in this confusing area of decision-making in dementia (Table 2.10)? Different countries and cultures have differing balances between the various principles. In Scotland paternalism is gradually being discredited but may revive. Autonomy is relatively in the ascendant, though there is a gradual appreciation of its limitations. Pseudo-autonomy, especially that based on prior preferences, will work up to a point, but must be viewed with a sceptical eye. The law is advancing slowly to fill gaps. But this advance may still be halted. Government is likely to be concerned that proposals such as those of the Scottish Law Commission are too expensive, too controversial (regarding advance directives for health care) and possibly too intrusive. The result is further consultation and the prospect of watered-down legal reform.

Consultation

In the meantime we need to look for and research best practice. In my own view dangers arise most readily when isolated individuals – the sufferer, an isolated carer, a single professional – make major decisions without reference to others. Where there are doubts about the capacity of the person with dementia to

Table 2.10 Decision-making

Paternalism
Autonomy
The Law
Pseudo-autonomy
Good practice guidelines
Case conference

decide, and no legal provision for the case, where there are disagreements about the best course of action, where there are significant risks in the situation there should be consultation between all involved, including the sufferer as far as possible (or represented by their advocate or information on their prior wishes), probably in some form of case conference (Table 2.11).

We need effective, fair conference decisions. Conferences should not allow bullies to dominate, they must allow a full discussion of rights and risks; there should be an opportunity for really creative discussions on possible solutions and finding ways round the problem. Every case conference should have a clear agenda and be clear about its authority and the authority of its members. It should have clear outcomes and a plan to review or reconvene, including clear plans for what happens if things do not work out as expected. There must be clear and agreed dispute resolution machinery between the agencies involved.

Such conferences have no legal authority in Scotland, but, if they are properly conducted, should be able to claim the authority of the professionals involved, the sensitive reference to the sufferer and his or her family, consensus and good practice. They are relatively expensive in time. In Scotland there are usually difficulties in ensuring the attendance of general practitioners who are crucial to many of these decisions. The emphasis in community care legislation on social work-centred care management and a local government reorganisation has in some places slowed or even reversed the progress of multi-agency working. However, the model makes sense for an illness which is so multi-factorial and complex. It seems most likely to bring balanced decisions based on full knowledge of the problem and its potential solutions and reflecting all the interests involved. Indeed a previous proposal for law reform, by Scottish Action on Dementia in 1986, envisaged a conference-style hearing system (on the model of Scotland's Children's Hearings) which would have legal powers to intervene or appoint guardians with variable powers in the various aspects

Table 2.11 Case conference

Patient and network of carers

Assessment of problem(s) to be solved

Choices available:

> To patient
>
> To carers
>
> Legal provisions

Risks and rights debate

Conclusions – action or inaction

Communication (and confidentiality)

Review

---

of an individual's case, to deal with difficult or contentious problems which could not be dealt with effectively by local informal case conference.

The law's role in relation to people with dementia is to ensure autonomy where that is reasonable, to set rules for the appointment of agents and to monitor the work they do on behalf of sufferers, to endorse informal arrangements where they are working if they are challenged, and to pick up the pieces when informal arrangements fail. Sadly it is not yet achieving this for people with dementia in Scotland and in many other countries.

Conclusion

In conclusion we need a system of substitute decision-making which reflects the problems of dementia (Table 2.2). Where a person cannot make decisions for his or herself reliably, someone else may have to fill that gap on the basis of the minimum necessary intervention. But gap fillers need monitoring and we need to be as sure as possible that they are committed to the true best interests of the sufferer and not solely driven by their own self-interest. A final comment is necessary, however. It is a sad reflection on the present state of dementia care that I must end by saying that the autonomous decisions of people with dementia, the well-meaning paternalistic decisions of carers, the good guesses of what I have called pseudo-autonomy, case conference decisions, the determinations of courts and the best laid schemes for law reform can all founder on the rocks of inadequate funding, inadequate resources and lack of political will, which have to be partly put down to public indifference to the plight of some of the most vulnerable people in our communities.

Chapter 3

Demography, Needs and Planning:
The Challenge of a Changing Population

David Gordon and Paul Spicker

Introduction

Planning for the needs of people with dementia requires baseline information in five areas: the number of people affected, their present circumstances, what needs they have, how their needs are currently met, and how all of these can be expected to change in the foreseeable future. This chapter provides an overview of this baseline information.

No distinction is made between different types of dementia in this chapter. Such distinctions are of clinical importance, and likely to become more so as the potential for therapeutic intervention increases, but are currently of little significance for service planning, which must cope with the consequences rather than the causes of dementia.

Information on the population with dementia and informal carers is often based on limited samples and may be valid only for the place where, and time when, they were conducted. To illustrate this chapter we have drawn upon recent broad-based surveys undertaken by ourselves and colleagues in Tayside (Angus and Dundee; Spicker *et al.* 1995) and epidemiological calculations for Scotland. Readers will need to judge whether these results are directly applicable to their own areas, and we have tried to provide the information in a form which facilitates this.

The number of people affected

There is wide variation in prevalence rates reported by different studies (Kay 1991). There are many contentious methodological issues (Black *et al.* 1990; Copeland 1990; Jagger *et al.* 1992). Much of the difficulty lies with marginal or 'mild' dementia (Brayne and Ames 1988; Burvill 1993; Dawe, Proctor and

Philpot 1992; Mowry and Burvill 1988). This often involves a level of impairment which does not markedly interfere with normal daily functioning but which appears as a below-threshold score on cognitive tests (Clarke *et al.* 1991; Henderson and Huppert 1984). Low scores can also be caused by low educational level, low socio-economic status, impaired physical health, other psychiatric illness, deafness or other factors affecting performance on tests which are unconnected with the presence or absence of dementia (Blessed 1989; Brayne and Calloway 1990; Burvill 1993; O'Connor, Pollitt and Treasure 1991; O'Connor *et al.* 1991a).

There are numerous dementia prevalence studies in the literature, and several syntheses have been published (Bond 1987; Henderson 1986; Hofman *et al.* 1991; Jorm, Korten and Henderson 1987; Kay 1991). The EURODEM (Hofman *et al.* 1991) synthesis has a number of advantages over previous syntheses. It used more explicit and rigorous criteria for including or excluding studies. It included only studies which involved individual examination of subjects. It excluded studies which omitted institutional populations: such omission can have a substantial impact on the numerator in a prevalence calculation. It presents results for detailed age–sex groups and in a form which can, if required, be used to calculate statistical confidence limits.

In application EURODEM provides a mid-range estimate, a little higher than the popular Jorm *et al.* (1987) estimate. In a study which screened all those aged 75+ in a Tayside town, the number of probable dementia sufferers identified was, after making a pro rata allowance for non-response, virtually identical to an estimate based on EURODEM (Carr 1992).

Dementia is very strongly age-related (Figure 3.1; Table 3.1). Of 58,500 people with dementia in Scotland in 1994, 32,300 (55 per cent) were aged 80 and over and a further 17,400 (30 per cent) were in their 70s (Figure 3.2). Only 2500 (4 per cent) were under the age of 60. Nearly two-thirds of sufferers are women,

Table 3.1: EURODEM prevalence rates:
Age–sex specific rate per 1000 population

	Age group							
	30–59	*60–64*	*65–69*	*70–74*	*75–79*	*80–84*	*85–89*	*90+*
Male	1.6	15.8	21.7	46.1	50.4	120.9	184.5	320.0
Female	0.9	4.7	11.0	38.6	6.7	135.0	227.6	328.2

Source: Hofman *et al.* (1991).

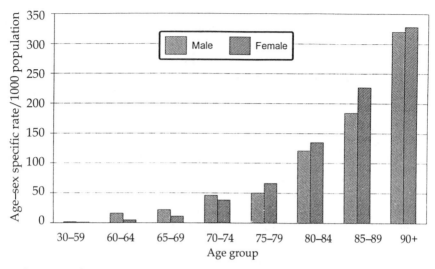

Source: Hofman *et al.* (1991)
Figure 3.1: Dementia prevalence rate by age and sex

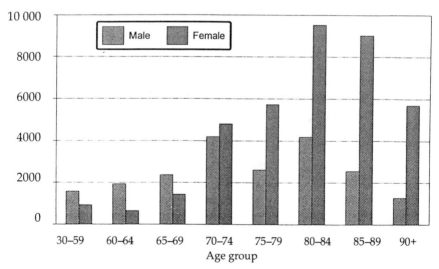

Source: Hofman *et al.* (1991) applied to Scottish population
Figure 3.2: Number of people with dementia by age and sex, Scotland 1994

reflecting the imbalance of the sexes in the elderly population. Because the problem of dementia is often reported in exaggerated tones, it is worth emphasising that only 1.1 per cent of the population of Scotland in 1994 had dementia, and 6.9 per cent of those aged 65 and over – substantial figures but hardly likely to bring about the collapse of civilisation as we know it.

There is little knowledge of the extent to which prevalence varies by locality (Blessed 1988), though recent research has found geographical variation in early onset Alzheimer's disease (Whalley *et al.* 1995) and local numbers can be distorted by the presence of large institutional populations (Martyn and Pippard 1988).

People with dementia are not the only ones affected by the disease. So too are families, friends and neighbours who care for them.

Caring often has its roots in the normal reciprocities of life and there is no universal definition of when someone is a 'carer' (Gordon and Donald 1993). There is little agreement between studies on the proportion of people with dementia in the community without an informal carer: 5 per cent (Badger, Cameron and Evers 1990), 18 per cent (McCullough 1980), 20–26 per cent (Levin, Sinclair and Gorbach 1983, 1989) and 34 per cent (Wenger 1994). In Tayside we found that around one in five of community residents with dementia apparently lacked an involved informal carer. The number of main informal carers in Scotland can be estimated thus:

- people aged 65+ with dementia   53,400
- 55 per cent of these are resident in the community   29,400
- of these 80 per cent have an informal carer   23,500

Assuming that most people under age 65 with dementia are resident in the community and that 80 per cent have an informal carer adds a further 4100 carers, giving around 28,000 main carers – 0.5 per cent of the population. More than one carer is not uncommon, though the balance of effort is rarely equal, so 28,000 is a minimum figure. Of course, this does not include those who maintain a significant and sometimes time-consuming commitment to caring about a relative who has been admitted to institutional care but who no longer have to bear the burden of caring directly *for* them.

The circumstances of people with dementia and informal carers

The idea that only a small minority of people with dementia live in institutional care (Jacques 1988) – residential and nursing homes and continuing care in hospitals – must be laid to rest (Preston 1986) (Table 3.2). Around 40 per cent

Table 3.2: Place of residence of people aged 65+ with dementia

	Tayside 1992–94		England 1985/86*
	Number	Per cent	Per cent
Ordinary housing	1339	45	}
Sheltered housing	341	11	} 63
Residential home – Local Authority	199	7	14
Residential home – private/voluntary	277	8	5
Nursing home	236	8	7
Psychogeriatric beds	314	10	}
Geriatric beds	347	12	} 11
Total	**3003**	**100**	**100**

* Kavanagh *et al.* (1993)

Table 3.3: Prevalence of dementia at age 65+ by place of residence

	Tayside: percentage of places/beds*	Published studies: percentage of residents**
Sheltered housing (dwellings)	7	–
Residential home – Local Authority	28	}
Residential home – private/voluntary	26	} 30–75
Nursing home	37	45–70
Long-stay geriatric	80	70–90
Psychogeriatric	70	80–90

*	Denominator data drawn from local statistical reports, particularly the Tayside Regional Council Community Care Plan, referring to various time periods.
**	See text for sources.

of sufferers are resident in institutions of various types. Although the proportion of people resident in long-term care will vary locally depending upon the level of institutional provision, for larger areas the greater variation is in the balance of care between different types of institution. For example, continuing hospital care for elderly people has been reduced faster in England than in

Scotland, with a correspondingly greater increase in residential and nursing home provision (Impallomenia and Starr 1995; Scottish Office 1995), though the total level of institutional provision in the two countries is roughly similar.

A wide range of prevalence of dementia has been reported from different institutional settings (Table 3.3) (Ames *et al.* 1988; *Bond 1987; Bond, Atkinson and Gregson 1989; Campbell, Crawford and Stout 1990; Campbell et al.* 1983; Clarke *et al.* 1991; de Zoysa and Blessed 1984; Donnelly *et al.* 1989; Gray *et al.* 1987; Ineichen 1990; Mann, Graham and Ashby 1984; O'Connor *et al.* 1989a; Preston 1986; Primrose and Capewell 1986; Shah *et al.* 1992; Williams *et al.* 1992).

Table 3.3 also shows our estimates for Tayside. These understate prevalence – perhaps by around one-tenth – since they are based on beds/places and not residents. The lower Tayside level in psychogeriatric beds possibly reflects the application of too strict a definition of dementia during data collection for the most specialist service. These qualifications do not explain the lower prevalence in Tayside residential and nursing homes compared with other studies. This is very likely to be a consequence of the relatively high level of institutional provision in Angus and Dundee: 189 and 152 beds/1000 population aged 75+ compared with a Scottish average of 135. This example shows very clearly how difficult it is to apply the results of published studies to a different area with any confidence.

Around one-half of people with dementia in the community known to services live with a carer (46 per cent in our Tayside surveys). A further few per cent live with a non-carer, usually a physically infirm spouse. In Tayside, where there is a high level of sheltered housing, half of those not living with an informal carer were in sheltered housing with a warden. People not known to services – which is about half of all those in the community with dementia (see below) – are as likely to have a co-resident carer as those known to services (Gordon 1994). As with most characteristics, results for co-residence vary between studies (Wenger 1994) because of both substantive and methodological differences.

It can be difficult for people with dementia to express themselves, especially as the disease progresses, and it is impossible to rely upon the factual accuracy of their statements, for example with regard to cooking abilities (Ballard *et al.* 1991). Hence most non-clinical studies and some clinical studies of dementia rely upon third parties – informal carers or professionals – as informants. Few samples of informal carers are representative (Barer and Johnson 1990; Baumgarten 1989; Dura and Kiecolt-Glaser 1990; Schulz, Visintainer and Williamson 1990). This is sometimes deliberate, for example with a decision to study only those who meet certain criteria, such as co-residence. Often, however, the bias comes with the use of a particular sampling frame, most notably in studies recruiting by self-selection or using samples from carer organisations and groups. Another significant source of bias can be refusal to participate in surveys.

One source of bias which has attracted criticism is that many studies have approached subjects through their pre-existing contact with services (Barer and Johnson 1990; Goodman 1986). However, surveys based upon the simultaneous censusing of a large number of services can minimise this problem at reasonable cost – around £8000 for a population of 270,000 (Gordon, Carter and Scott 1995).

One-fifth of people with dementia in the community who are known to services lack an informal carer, approaching half have a co-resident carer and one-third have an informal carer who lives elsewhere but who visits. Of the 80 per cent with a carer, two-thirds have one carer, one-fifth two carers, and only one-tenth have three or more carers to share the burden.

That caring work falls disproportionately to women is well known (Parker 1990), though with increasing acknowledgement of the importance of older male spouses as carers (Fisher 1994). In Tayside, 69 per cent of main carers were women, as were 62 per cent of second and 69 per cent of third carers. The relationship of the main carer to the sufferer was: daughter 34 per cent, wife 23 per cent, husband 13 per cent, son 13 per cent, other relative 13 per cent, and friend/neighbour 3 per cent. Many carers are themselves elderly (Arber and Ginn 1990; Wenger 1990): in Tayside two-fifths of main carers were aged 65 or older and one-fifth were aged 75 or over. Only one-quarter were under age 50.

The needs of people with dementia and informal carers

Planning for the needs of a population with dementia requires a broad-brush understanding of needs. The detail required in individual assessment (Hughes 1993; McWalter *et al.* 1994) is unhelpful at the planning level. It is expensive and complex to collect through surveys; liable to reflect levels of demand for current services if collected through routine assessments; and in any case it is impossible to plan services to such a degree of detail or to deliver them with sufficient timing for the detail still to be applicable as the population changes constantly. Matching the detail of needs and services for the individual is the province of professional practice. However, neither is a simple numerical approach to needs appropriate without differentiation between different types and levels of need. The more useful dependency measures are those which use descriptive categories rather than numerical scores (Wilkin and Thompson 1989).

The Tayside profile uses the time interval for which the sufferer can manage without assistance to identify level of need in respect of mobility, personal care, domestic tasks and behaviour. Before describing needs, we need to digress briefly to describe the survey data with which we illustrate this section. Multi-service censuses (Gordon *et al.* 1993) in Angus and Dundee identified 2238 of an expected 3003 individuals, based on EURODEM prevalence, reduced to 2163 after elimination of false positives. Data on needs indicators were obtained for a sample of 805 individuals with dementia, and for informal carers where appropriate, with informants being institutional staff (499), community profes-sionals (115) and informal carers (191). Those not identified by a service census have, on average, less cognitive and physical impairment, greater inde-pendence in activities of daily living, lower service use and less carer burden (Gordon 1994).

There is a general progression in the time interval needs of people with dementia across care settings offering different levels of care (Table 3.4). But what is no less striking is the high level of critical and short-interval needs in community settings. Applying the proportions in Table 3.4 to the estimated number of people with dementia known to services in different settings (which we consider below) shows, for example, that in Tayside there were 250 people in the community with critical interval need for attention because of behav-ioural problems compared with 216 in geriatric continuing care and only 44 in local authority residential care. Putting it another way, 28 per cent of the estimated 893 people with behaviour-related critical interval need were living in the community.

We found, contrary to expectation, a generally lower level of need in sheltered housing than in mainstream housing. This might arise from the high level of provision of sheltered housing locally. But it also raises questions about the level of need which can be accommodated in conventional sheltered hous-ing (Sinclair *et al.* 1990).

Another aspect of need is the need for social interaction. In Tayside, 14 per cent of community-resident sufferers were normally alone for more than ten hours during the day (not counting any time spent alone overnight) and a further 26 per cent usually spent 5–10 hours alone.

In common with the elderly population as a whole, dementia sufferers have material needs. Eighteen per cent of community residents lived in housing deficient in sanitation, lacking central heating or in need of major repair. The sole source of income for 24 per cent of sufferers was the state pension; a further 39 per cent had additional income only from state disability or carer benefits.

Table 3.4: Need for assistance with mobility, personal care, domestic tasks and behaviour by place of residence, Tayside, 1992–94

Column percentage

Type of need Interval of need	Community	Local Authority residential home	Private/ voluntary residential home	Nursing home	Psychiatric continuing care	Geriatric continuing care
Mobility						
Independent	62	50	34	23	15	0
Long interval	16	34	21	16	21	2
Short interval	14	9	25	47	34	50
Critical interval	8	7	20	14	30	48
Personal care						
Independent	38	19	15	2	0	1
Long interval	22	38	23	21	8	1
Short interval	18	24	19	28	26	19
Critical interval	22	18	43	48	66	78
Personal care – night						
No help needed	77	72	38	33	16	2
Help needed	23	28	62	67	84	98
Domestic tasks						
Independent	7	10	6	0	0	1
Long interval	27	34	10	12	3	0
Short interval	66	56	84	88	97	99
Behaviour						
Independent	26	28	16	15	4	9
Long interval	19	35	22	13	10	10
Short interval	25	16	17	28	30	19
Critical interval	34	22	46	44	56	62
Behaviour – night						
No help needed	82	70	46	39	24	26
Help needed	18	30	54	61	76	74
Sample number (=100%)	184–189	92–110	68–88	75–105	67–103	87–93

Key:
Independent – attention needed less than once a week.
Long interval – attention needed not more than once a day.
Short interval – attention needed more than once a day at pre-arranged times.
Critical interval – intervention needed more than once a day at unpredictable or very frequent (less than 2 hour) intervals.

Only 37 per cent had a private income, including 15 per cent who also had disability/carer benefits.

A very important component of a population needs assessment for dementia is the burden placed upon informal carers. There can be rewards as well as burdens from caring (Levin *et al.* 1989), but it is the burdens for which services must plan. The literature on the impact of caring upon carers is extensive, though frequently flawed by inadequate samples, as we have already noted. (A useful short summary is Kruse (1991).) Both objective and subjective components are involved in the response of carers to caring (Duijnstee 1992, 1994; Orbell, Hopkins and Gillies 1993). In Tayside, for example, more than two-fifths (44 per cent) of carers had practical problems in caring and half (52 per cent) were experiencing emotional upset. Despite this only a small minority of carers (14 per cent) were failing to cope with caring.

Support to carers who wish to continue is essential, but so too is recognition that some relationships cannot sustain the trials of caring (Gilhooly *et al.* 1994; Motenko 1989; Wenger 1990). Over time the burden of caring can become too great even for the most committed carer and many dementia sufferers end their days in settings designed for the professional provision of 24 hour care. Admission to such 'terminal care' (Philp *et al.* in preparation) should not be viewed as a bad outcome: the evidence suggests that it may be unavoidable (Gilhooly 1990; Melzer *et al.* 1992; O'Connor *et al.* 1991b).

Table 3.5: People aged 65+ with dementia known to services by place of residence, Tayside 1992–94

	Number	*Per cent*
Housing (mainstream/sheltered)	840	39
Residential home – Local Authority	199	9
Residential home – private/voluntary	227	10
Nursing home	236	11
Psychogeriatric beds	314	15
Geriatric beds	347	16
Total	**2163**	**100**

How are needs currently met?

The majority of people with dementia are known to services (Livingston *et al.* 1990; O'Connor *et al.* 1989b). In Tayside the censuses of those known to services as having problems symptomatic of dementia identified 72 per cent of the number expected from the EURODEM prevalence estimate, after eliminating false positives (Table 3.5). On the assumption that all those not known to services are resident in the community, exactly half of the expected number of people with dementia in the community were known to services. Another Scottish survey found 78 per cent known to services and 53 per cent in the community (Gordon *et al.* 1995).

A point of particular importance is that no one service or agency provides the key to identifying people with dementia (Table 3.6). General practice is the most important single community source, though the inconclusive literature on the extent to which GPs know of dementia sufferers on their lists suggests that local variation might be substantial (Iliffe *et al.* 1990; Ineichen 1989; Levin *et al.* 1989; O'Connor *et al.* 1988; Philp and Young 1988). (The high level for sheltered housing wardens in Table 3.7 reflects Tayside's high level of provision.)

The services potentially available are well reviewed by Melzer *et al.* (1992). The particular level of provision of services and the balance between different services depends upon local policies. There is ample evidence that service inputs to the non-institutional care of people with dementia are surprisingly low, even among those identified through contact with services (Levin *et al.* 1989; O'Connor *et al.* 1989b; Philp *et al.* 1995; Schneider *et al.* 1993; Wenger 1994). At the time of our Tayside surveys, provision of domiciliary and day services taken as a whole was somewhat below the Scottish average, and Tables 3.7 and 3.8, showing services used by those known to services, must be viewed in that light. The importance of home help, district nurse, general practitioner and day services is clearly seen in Table 3.7. If the backbone of community care is informal carers, then the primary ribs are the home help and district nursing services. In addition to the services shown, 25 per cent of sufferers had received residential or inpatient respite care within the past year. Service use by those not known to services is likely to be substantially lower (Gordon 1994; Wenger 1994).

In developing the Tayside profile we could not measure the input of community services on the 'interval' basis we used for needs, because only rarely are services actually provided at critical or even short interval intensity. This is in marked contrast to the level of support provided by informal carers. In Tayside, 53 per cent of dementia sufferers in the community had short or critical

Table 3.6: Service returns to censuses, Tayside 1992–94

Percentage of individuals identified by each service*

	All returns		Community residents	
	Total	Sole source	Total	Sole source
Community health				
GP	26	16	32	26
District nurse	7	2	13	6
Continence adviser	6	3	4	2
Chiropody	5	3	7	6
Day hospital	4	1	9	3
Health visitor	1	1	2	1
Community psychiatric nurse	1	0	2	1
Community social				
Sheltered housing	11	10	27	26
Home help	10	6	23	14
Social worker	10	5	15	8
Day care**	4	2	9	4
Occupational therapy	2	1	2	0
Voluntary/carer groups	4	1	6	1
Medical and care establishments				
Residential home	19	16	0	0
Psychiatric	14	15	0	0
Geriatric	11	12	1	1
Nursing home	7	5	0	0
Physiotherapy	3	1	0	0
Total persons (=100%)	2238	1563	917	628

*   Columns for totals sum to more than 100% because of multiple returns for individuals.

**   Includes voluntary day care.

Table 3.7: Frequency of receipt of main community services by people aged 65+ with dementia, Tayside 1992–94*

Row percentage

| | *Number of days received in past 28 days* | | | | | | |
	0	1	2–3	4	5–8	9–16	17–28
Home help	42	1	2	15	15	6	17
District nurse	62	5	10	8	4	2	10
General practitioner	69	20	9	1	<0.5	<0.5	0
Day care	72	1	3	7	8	6	4
Day hospital	83	<0.5	<0.5	6	6	3	1
Meals on wheels	87	<0.5	<0.5	3	8	2	<0.5
Social worker	88	7	3	1	<0.5	<0.5	<0.5

*   Includes services received by carers specifically to help with caring.
         Sample number = 306.

Table 3.8: Receipt of less common community services by people aged 65+ with dementia, Tayside 1992–94*

	Percentage receiving service in past 28 days
Day sitter	9
Laundry	7
Occupational therapist	5
Community psychiatric nurse	5
Continence adviser	4
Lunch club	3
Carers group	3
Health visitor	2
Night sitter	<0.5

*   Includes services received by carers specifically to help with caring.
         Sample number = 306.

Table 3.9: Informal care inputs, Tayside 1992–94

Percentage Interval of input*	Mainstream housing	Sheltered housing	Total community
Daytime			
Independent	8	11	9
Long interval	23	36	28
Short interval	19	23	20
Critical interval	50	30	43
Night			
No help needed	57	82	66
Help needed	43	18	34
Sample number (=100%)	164–169	91–98	255–367

*   Columns for totals sum to more than 100% because of multiple returns for individuals.

interval intervention by informal carers, while only 10 per cent had home help daily. The level of informal care input differed markedly between mainstream and sheltered housing in Tayside, in part because of the greater proportion of co-resident carers in mainstream housing (Table 3.9). (Levels of needs were also lower in sheltered housing but not so markedly.) If informal carers did not exist, the whole policy of care in the community – insofar as it means care in people's own homes – would collapse.

Despite the importance of informal care and policies which are intended to encourage the support of people in their own homes, the bulk of expenditure on people with dementia is on institutional care (Kavanagh *et al*. 1993; Schneider *et al*. 1993). This applies whether the opportunity costs of informal care are included or not.

The future

Information about the current status quo is usually the best information available from which to determine the potential pattern of a population's needs in the future. However, the cohort whose needs is identified at one point in time is not necessarily that for which resources will be provided at a future point.

Table 3.10: Deaths and removals, people aged 65+ with dementia, Tayside 1991–94; Forth Valley 1995

Percentage of operational sample

	Angus	Dundee	Forth Valley
Dead	14.8	8.8	4.5
Transferred to institutional care/moved	15.8	13.4	7.6
Total losses	30.6	22.2	12.1
Operational sample (n = 100%)	609	758	422
Mean follow-up (days)	231	123	70

This is particularly true of the population with dementia, which demonstrates extremely high levels of residential relocation and death (Table 3.10). This is well known to those responsible for the care of individuals since it creates much difficulty in the organisation of care packages. The flow of people through a constantly changing population pool also has implications for higher level planning.

There are three main flows in the population with dementia:

• inflow by incidence and immigration

• transfers between community and institutional residence

• outflow by mortality and emigration.

Estimates of incidence depend greatly on the definition of the disease, with the greatest uncertainty concerning those categorised as mild dementia. Published rates vary widely: for example, 9.2 per 1000 aged 65 and over in Liverpool (Copeland *et al.* 1992) and Nottingham (Morgan *et al.* 1993); 15.4 in Germany (Bickel and Cooper 1994); 16.3 in France (Letenneur *et al.* 1994); and 26 in London (Boothby *et al.* 1994). A more recent study has suggested a rate of only 9.2 per 1000 aged 75 and over (Brayne *et al.* 1995). Differences are caused by methodological differences and difficulties: incidence and prevalence rates have shown no change in the past few decades (Kay 1991).

The available information on mortality is also limited. Published data show annualised rates of around 20–30 per cent (Copeland *et al.* 1992; Gilleard 1985). Returns from the Tayside censuses suggested an annual mortality rate in the range of 23–26 per cent. This may be an underestimate because of possible unidentified mortality among those moving to institutional care. However, since cases known to services are more impaired their death rate will be higher than for the total population with dementia. The population annual mortality rate may be around 20 per cent. From data in Opit and Pahl (1993) a community annual mortality rate of 12 per cent for those aged 75 and over can be estimated. Mortality is substantially higher among those in institutional care than in the community (Ballinger *et al.* 1988; Bowling, Formby and Grant 1993; Shah *et al.* 1993).

A simple way of estimating incidence is to assume that it is unchanging and therefore that it must balance out deaths. In an ageing population, the number of new cases of dementia will be greater than loss due to mortality. If annual mortality is, say, 20 per cent then incidence must be 20 per cent plus an increment from population change.

The incidence of permanent institutional admission of people with dementia appears to be high, though many samples are of extreme populations such as psychogeriatric referrals (Gilleard 1985; Goda 1985; Jerrom, Mian and Rukanyake 1993; Knopman *et al.* 1988). In our Angus census 77 people out of 278 had moved to institutions in a 231 day period, suggesting an annual movement of 43 per cent. In the Dundee census 75 people out of 398 transferred to institutional care in a 123 day period, suggesting a higher annual rate of 56 per cent. This may be an overstatement since not all those entering hospital could confidently be identified as having made a permanent move. Nonetheless, 40–50 per cent of those in the community *recognised to have dementia* may move to institutions in the course of a year.

This is a substantial overestimate for the total population with dementia. If sufferers in the community not known to services experience a 10 per cent rate of admission, the admission rate for the total community population with dementia would be 25 per cent. This is plausible since some of those not known to services are being 'shielded' by an informal carer and will only come to the attention of services when a crisis in their condition or their care triggers an urgent admission to institutional care. However, it is higher than Opit and Pahl's (1993) estimate of 21 per cent for those aged 75 and over.

Information on the migration patterns of people with dementia is totally lacking. Detailed longitudinal information about transfers of people with dementia between different institutional settings is also extremely limited (Ashby *et al.* 1991; Marshall 1994).

It is possible to model the flow of the population aged 65 and over with dementia in Scotland for the next 15 years. The model is based on the following assumptions:

- Total prevalence is calculated by applying EURODEM to General Register Office (Scotland) population projections.

- In any year, incidence is 20 per cent of the existing population with dementia (i.e. equivalent to mortality) plus the difference between that year's and the previous year's total prevalence. Ninety per cent of incidence is assumed to be in the community and 10 per cent in institutions. (Setting 'replacement' incidence at 20% is equivalent to a rate of 15 per 1000 aged 65 and over in the current Scottish population.)

- In any year mortality is 20 per cent of the population with dementia. This is a 9 per cent rate for the population in the community and a 33 per cent rate in the institutional population. Net migration is assumed to be nil.

- The initial balance of care between community and institutional residence is set at 55:45. The annual rate of transfer from community to institutions is 25 per cent.

Table 3.11: Modelling the future flow of people aged 65+ with dementia, Scotland 1995–2010

	Total prevalence	Total incidence	Total mortality	Community prevalence*	Transfers: community to institutional	Institutional prevalence*
1995	55,183	11,880	11,037	30,588	7647	24,702
2000	58,742	12,634	11,748	32,106	8004	26,884
2005	62,324	13,295	12,465	33,823	8456	28,548
2010	66,104	14,126	13,221	35,857	8964	30,252

*   Community and institutional prevalence do not sum to the total prevalence because the model is not exact.

The resulting model of annual flows is summarised in Table 3.11. This assumes that the present balance between institutional and community residence is maintained. Anecdotal evidence suggests this is so far the case: 'care in the community' for people with dementia has meant the replacement of hospital beds by nursing home beds rather than greater care for people at home. The data and assumptions underlying this model cannot be applied to the population under age 65 in which incidence, mortality and institutionalisation rates are lower (McGonigal *et al.* 1993; Newens, Forster and Kay 1995).

On the basis of these assumptions – and planning is largely the business of making and testing different assumptions about what the future might look like – by 2010 there will be 66,100 people aged 65 and over with dementia (plus 5800 under the age of 65). Nearly 36,000 will live in the community, an increase

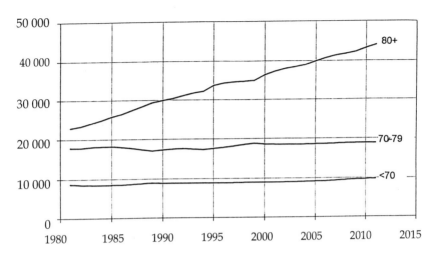

Source: Hofman *et al.* (1991) applied to Scottish population estimates and projections
Figure 3.3 Trend in number of people with dementia by age, Scotland

of 6500 on 1994, and just over 30,000 in institutions, an increase of 6200. The increase in institutional care might be greater than this if the current criteria for institutional admission are maintained, since almost all of the increase will be in the very elderly population, as it has been for the past decade (Figure 3.3). The scale of change required to alter the balance of community and institutional care is striking. To reduce the proportion in institutions from 45 per cent to 35 per cent requires a sustained reduction of 40 per cent in the annual transfer rate (from 25% to 15%).

Using the same assumptions as in the model, it can be shown that a cohort of people with dementia in the community will be reduced to only 12 per cent of its original number in five years, while a cohort in institutional care will be reduced to 14 per cent of its original number. It is possible to vary the assumptions to test, for example, the effect of a higher or lower mortality rate on cohort survival. This has little impact on the Scottish projections since they are controlled by the population projections. At the national scale, if we assume higher (or lower) mortality we have to build in higher (or lower) incidence to compensate, since we have an independent projection of the total prevalence for each year.

In building this simple spreadsheet model we have had to make explicit assumptions that can often remain hidden and implicit within the planning process. The key message is that the 'population' with dementia for whom plans are being made is a transient one, with an estimated one-third changing circumstances radically each year through death or institutional admission. The population of carers also shows a high degree of volatility (Taylor, Ford and Dunbar 1995). Given the time lag between population needs assessment and service developments, the population for whom new services are implemented seldom matches the population whose needs were assessed. Hence there is only a limited advantage in trying to develop highly accurate and detailed data in relation to problems which cannot be responded to immediately. Greater precision in assessing needs in the current cohort may even be misleading since it does not necessarily mean greater precision in *anticipating* the needs of the future population.

There is also an important issue for policy and practice. People who have dementia over a long period of time in stable circumstances are untypical. Services need to be geared to providing responses for relatively short periods, and to be sufficiently flexible to respond to changes in circumstances. No service can achieve this in isolation and a nominated 'key contact' may be critical in enabling continuity of care to be maintained.

Conclusion

Planning for populations and planning for individuals are two quite different activities. The preoccupation of those planning for populations with numbers, projections and the provenance and robustness of assumptions does not sit easily with the concern of professionals in the caring services with the uniqueness of the quality of life of each individual. Yet seeking to capture the uniqueness of the individual is positively counter-productive for planning. Precision in establishing the needs of the current population is less important than ensuring that the services which are planned and provided are robust enough – 'future-proofed' – to cope with changes in the pattern of needs which will inevitably occur as successive cohorts age. This requires flexibility not merely in a few special projects but throughout mainstream services. The challenge that must be met by planners is the creation of frameworks that enable and encourage the provision of services that are flexible and responsive to individual need in both domestic and institutional settings.

References

Ames, D., Ashby, D., Mann, A.H. and Graham, N. (1988) 'Psychiatric illness in elderly residents in Part III homes in one London borough: prognosis and review.' *Age and Ageing 17*, 249–256.

Arber, S. and Ginn, J. (1990) 'The meaning of informal care: gender and the contribution of elderly people.' *Ageing and Society 10*, 429–454.

Ashby, D., Ames, D., West, C.R., MacDonald, A., Graham, N. and Mann, A.H. (1991) 'Psychiatric morbidity as predictor of mortality for residents of local authority homes for the elderly.' *International Journal of Geriatric Psychiatry 6*, 567–575.

Badger, F., Cameron, E. and Evers, H. (1990) 'Waiting to be served/slipping through the net.' *Health Service Journal*, 11 Jan./18 Jan., 54–55, 86–87.

Ballard, C.G., Chithiramohan, R.N., Handy, S., Bannister, C., Davis, R. and Todd, N.B. (1991) 'Information reliability in dementia sufferers.' *International Journal of Geriatric Psychiatry 6*, 313–316.

Ballinger, B.R., McHarg, A.M., MacLennan, W.J. and Ogston, S. (1988) 'Dementia psychiatric symptoms and immobility: a one-year follow-up.' *International Journal of Geriatric Psychiatry 3*, 125–129.

Barer, B.M. and Johnson, C.L. (1990) 'A critique of the caregiving literature.' *Gerontologist 30*, 26–29.

Baumgarten, M. (1989) 'The health of persons giving care to the demented elderly: a critical review of the literature.' *Journal of Clinical Epidemiology 42*, 1137–1148.

Bickel, H. and Cooper, B. (1994) 'Incidence and relative risk of dementia in an urban elderly population.' *Psychological Medicine 24*, 179–192.

Black, S., Blessed, G., Edwardson, J. and Kay, D. (1990) 'Prevalence rates of dementia in an ageing population: are low rates due to the use of insensitive instruments?' *Age and Ageing 19*, 84–90.

Blessed, G. (1988) 'Long stay beds for the elderly severely mentally ill: a discussion paper.' *Bulletin of the Royal College of Psychiatrists 12*, 250–252.

Blessed, G. (1989) 'Definition and classification of the dementias: the point of view of a clinician.' In J. Wertheimer, P. Baumann, M. Gaillard and P. Schwed (eds) *Innovative Trends in Psychogeriatrics*. Basel: Karger.

Bond, J. (1987) 'Psychiatric illness in later life: a study of prevalence in a Scottish population.' *International Journal of Geriatric Psychiatry 2*, 39–57.

Bond, J., Atkinson, A. and Gregson, B.A. (1989) 'The prevalence of psychiatric illness among continuing-care patients under the care of departments of geriatric medicine.' *International Journal of Geriatric Psychiatry 4*, 227–233.

Boothby, H., Blizard, R., Livingston, G. and Mann, A. (1994) 'The Gospel Oak Study stage III: the incidence of dementia.' *Psychological Medicine 24*, 89–95.

Bowling, A., Formby, J. and Grant, K. (1993) 'Factors associated with mortality in national health service nursing homes for elderly people and long-stay geriatric wards in hospital.' *International Journal of Geriatric Psychiatry 8*, 203–210.

Brayne, C. and Ames, D. (1988) 'The epidemiology of mental illness in old age.' In B. Gearing, M. Johnson and T. Heller (eds) *Mental Health Problems in Old Age.* Chichester: Wiley.

Brayne, C. and Calloway, P. (1990) 'The association of education and socio-economic status with the Mini-Mental State Examination and the clinical diagnosis of dementia in elderly people.' *Age and Ageing 19*, 91–96.

Brayne, C., Gill, C., Huppert, F.A., Barkley, C., Gelhaar, E., Girling, D.M., O'Connor, D.W. and Paykel, E.S. (1995) 'Incidence of clinically diagnosed subtypes of dementia in an elderly population.' *British Journal of Psychiatry 167*, 255–262.

Burvill, P.W. (1993) 'A critique of current criteria for early dementia in epidemiological studies.' *International Journal of Geriatric Psychiatry 8*, 553–559.

Campbell, A.J., McCosh, L.M., Reinken, J. and Allan, B.C. (1983) 'Dementia in old age and the need for services.' *Age and Ageing 12*, 11–16.

Campbell, H., Crawford, V. and Stout, R.W. (1990) 'The impact of private residential and nursing care on statutory residential and hospital care of elderly people in south Belfast.' *Age and Ageing 19*, 318–324.

Carr, J. (1992) *Tayside Dementia Services Planning Survey.* Stirling: Dementia Services Development Centre, University of Stirling.

Clarke, M., Jagger, C., Anderson, J., Battcock, T., Kelly, F. and Stern, M.C. (1991) 'The prevalence of dementia in a total population: a comparison of two screening instruments.' *Age and Ageing 20*, 396–403.

Copeland, J.R.M. (1990) 'Suitable instruments for detecting dementia in community samples.' *Age and Ageing 19*, 81–83.

Copeland, J.R.M., Davidson, I.A., Dewey, M.E., Gilmore, C., Larkin, B.A., McWilliam, C., Saunders, P.A., Scott, A., Sharma, V. and Sullivan, C. (1992) 'Alzheimer's disease, other dementias, depression and pseudodementia: prevalence, incidence and three-year outcome in Liverpool.' *British Journal of Psychiatry 161*, 230–239.

Dawe, B., Proctor, A. and Philpot, M. (1992) 'Concepts of mild memory impairment in the elderly and their relationship to dementia: a review.' *International Journal of Geriatric Psychiatry 7*, 473–479.

de Zoysa, A.S.R. and Blessed, G. (1984) 'The place of the specialist home for the elderly mentally infirm in the care of mentally disturbed old people.' *Age and Ageing 13*, 218–223.

Donnelly, C.M., Compton, S.A., Devany, N., Kirk, S. and McGuigan, M. (1989) 'The elderly in long term care: 1 – prevalence of dementia and levels of dependency.' *International Journal of Geriatric Psychiatry 4*, 299–304.

Duijnstee, M. (1992) 'Caring for demented family members at home: objective observation and subjective evaluation of burden.' In G.M.M. Jones and B.M.L. Miesen (eds) *Care-Giving in Dementia: Research and Applications.* London: Routledge.

Duijnstee, M.S.H. (1994) 'Relatives of persons suffering from dementia: differences in the burden.' *Ageing and Society 14*, 499–519.

Dura, J.R. and Kiecolt-Glaser, J.K. (1990) 'Sample bias in caregiving research.' *Journal of Gerontology 45*, P200–P204.

Fisher, M. (1994) 'Man-made care: community care and older male carers.' *British Journal of Social Work 24*, 659–680.

Gilhooly, M.L.M. (1990) *Do Services Delay or Prevent Institutionalisation of People with Dementia?* Stirling: Dementia Services Development Centre, University of Stirling.

Gilhooly, M.L.M., Sweeting, H.N., Whittick, J.E. and McKee, K. (1994) 'Family care of the dementing elderly.' *International Review of Psychiatry 6*, 29–40.

Gilleard, C.J. (1985) 'The impact of psychogeriatric day care on the patient's supporting relatives.' *Health Bulletin 43*, 199–205.

Goda, D. (1985) *Pathways into and between services for the elderly in Scotland.* Unpublished report to Scottish Home and Health Department.

Goodman, C. (1986) 'Research on the informal carer: a selected literature review.' *Journal of Advanced Nursing 11*, 705–712.

Gordon, D.S. (1994) Unpublished reanalysis of original data from Carr (1992). Anonymous data kindly supplied by Dementia Services Development Centre, University of Stirling.

Gordon, D.S. and Donald, S.C. (1993) *Community Social Work, Older People and Informal Care.* Aldershot: Avebury.

Gordon, D.S., Gillies, B., McWilliam, N. and Spicker, P. (1993) 'A local census of dementia sufferers.' *Scottish Medical Journal 386*, 186–187.

Gordon, D.S., Carter, H. and Scott, S. (1995) *The Needs of Elderly People with Problems of Memory/Confusion: Survey Report.* Stirling: Forth Valley Health Board.

Gray, R.F., Hughes, A.M., Downie, D., Hohiuddin, A. and Hall, W.S. (1987) 'Long-term care for the elderly – who goes where?' *Health Bulletin 45*, 11–14.

Henderson, A.S. (1986) 'The epidemiology of Alzheimer's Disease.' *British Medical Journal 42*, 3–10.

Henderson, A.S. and Huppert, F.A. (1984) 'The problem of mild dementia.' *Psychological Medicine 14*, 5–11.

Hofman, A., Rocca, W.A., Brayne, C., Breteler, M.M.B. *et al.* (1991) 'The prevalence of dementia in Europe: a collaborative study of 1980–1990 findings.' *International Journal of Epidemiology 20*, 736–748.

Hughes, B. (1993) 'A model for the comprehensive assessment of older people and their carers.' *British Journal of Social Work 23*, 345–364.

Iliffe, S., Booroff, A., Gallivan, S., Goldenberg, E., Morgan, P. and Haines, A. (1990) 'Screening for cognitive impairment in the elderly using the mini-mental state examination.' *British Journal of General Practice 40*, 277–279.

Impallomenia, M. and Starr, J. (1995) 'The changing face of community and institutional care for the elderly.' *Journal of Public Health Medicine 17*, 171–178.

Ineichen, B. (1989) *Senile Dementia: Policy and Services.* London: Chapman and Hall.

Ineichen, B. (1990) 'The extent of dementia among old people in residential care.' *International Journal of Geriatric Psychiatry 5*, 327–335.

Jacques, A. (1988) *Understanding Dementia*. Edinburgh: Churchill Livingston.

Jagger, C., Clarke, M., Anderson, J. and Battcock, T. (1992) 'Dementia in Melton Mowbray: a validation of earlier findings.' *Age and Ageing 21*, 205–210.

Jerrom, B., Mian, I. and Rukanyake, N.G. (1993) 'Stress on relative caregivers of dementia sufferers and predictors of breakdown of community care.' *International Journal of Geriatric Psychiatry 8*, 331–337.

Jorm, A.F., Korten, A.E. and Henderson, A.S. (1987) 'The prevalence of dementia: a quantitative integration of the literature.' *Acta Psychiatrica Scandinavica 76*, 465–479.

Kavanagh, S., Schneider, J., Knapp, M., Neechman, J. and Netten, A. (1993) 'Elderly people with cognitive impairment: costing possible changes in the balance of care.' *Health and Social Care 1*, 69–80.

Kay, D.W.K. (1991) 'The epidemiology of dementia: a review of recent work.' *Reviews in Clinical Gerontology 1*, 55–66.

Knopman, D., Kitto, J., Deinard, S. and Heiring, J. (1988) 'Longitudinal study of death and institutionalisation in patients with primary degenerative disorder.' *Journal of the American Geriatrics Society 36*, 108–112.

Kruse, A. (1991) 'Caregivers coping with chronic disease, dying and death of an aged family.' *Reviews in Clinical Gerontology 1*, 411–415.

Letenneur, L., Commenges, D., Dartigues, J.F. and Barberger-Gateau, P. (1994) 'Incidence of dementia and Alzheimer's Disease in elderly community residents of south-western France.' *International Journal of Epidemiology 23*, 1256–1261.

Levin, E., Sinclair, I. and Gorbach, P. (1983) *The Supporters of Confused Elderly Persons at Home, Vol 3: Appendices*. London: National Institute for Social Work.

Levin, E., Sinclair, I. and Gorbach, P. (1989) *Families, Services and Confusion in Old Age*. Aldershot: Avebury.

Livingstone, G., Thomas, A., Graham, N., Blizard, B. and Mann, A. (1990) 'The Gospel Oak Project: The use of health and social sciences by dependent elderly people in the community.' *Health Trends 22*, 70–73.

Mann, A.H., Graham, N. and Ashby, D. (1984) 'Psychiatric illness in residential homes for the elderly: a survey of one London borough.' *Age and Ageing 13*, 257–265.

Marshall, M. (1994) *A Home for Life? Profiling of People with Dementia for Long-Stay Care*. Edinburgh: Scottish Action on Dementia.

Martyn, C.N. and Pippard, E.C. (1988) 'Usefulness of mortality data in determining the geography and time trends of dementia.' *Journal of Epidemiology and Community Health 42*, 134–37.

McCullough, D.R. (1980) *The Needs of Carers of Elderly People with Dementia*. Glasgow: Strathclyde Regional Council.

McGonigal, G., Thomas, B., McQuade, C., Starr, J.M., MacLennan, W.J. and Whalley, L.J. (1993) 'Epidemiology of Alzheimer's presenile dementia in Scotland, 1974-88.' *British Medical Journal 306*, 680–683.

McWalter, G., Toner, H., Corser, A., Eastwood, J., Marshall, M. and Turvey, T. (1994) 'Needs and needs assessment: their components and definitions with reference to dementia.' *Health and Social Care 2*, 213–219.

Melzer, D., Hopkins, S., Pencheon, D., Brayne, C. and Williams, R. (1992) *Epidemiologically Based Needs Assessment: Dementia.* London: NHS Management Executive.

Morgan, K., Lilley, J.M., Arie, T., Byrne, E.J., Jones, R. and Waite, J. (1993) 'Incidence of dementia in a representative British sample.' *British Journal of Psychiatry 163*, 467–470.

Motenko, A.K. (1989) 'The frustrations, gratifications and well-being of dementia caregivers.' *The Gerontologist 29*, 166–172.

Mowry, B.J. and Burvill, P.W. (1988) 'A study of mild dementia in the community using a wide range of diagnostic criteria.' *British Journal of Psychiatry 153*, 328–334.

Newens, A.J., Forster, D.P. and Kay, D.W.K. (1995) 'Dependency and community care in pre-senile Alzheimer's Disease.' *British Journal of Psychiatry 166*, 777–782.

O'Connor, D.W., Pollitt, P.A., Hyde, J.B., Brook, C.P.B., Reiss, B.B. and Roth, M. (1988) 'Do general practitioners miss dementia in elderly patients?' *British Medical Journal 297*, 1107–1110.

O'Connor, D.W., Pollitt, P.A., Hyde, J.B., Fellows, J.L., Miller, N.D., Brook, C.P.B., Reiss, B.B. and Roth, M. (1989a) 'The prevalence of dementia as measured by the Cambridge Mental Disorders of the Elderly Examination.' *Acta Psychiatrica Scandinavica 79*, 190–198.

O'Connor, D.W., Pollitt, P.A., Brook, C.P.B. and Reiss, B.B. (1989b) 'The distribution of services to demented elderly people living in the community.' *International Journal of Geriatric Psychiatry 4*, 339–344.

O'Connor, D.W., Pollitt, P.A., Hyde, J.B., Fellowes, J.L., Miller, N.D. and Roth, M. (1991a) 'The progression of mild idiopathic dementia in a community population.' *Journal of the American Geriatrics Society 39*, 246–251.

O'Connor, D.W., Pollitt, P.A., Brook, C.P.B., Reiss, B.B. and Roth, M. (1991b) 'Does early intervention reduce the number of elderly people with dementia admitted to institutions for long term care? *British Medical Journal 302*, 871–875.

O'Connor, D.W., Pollitt, P. and Treasure, F.P. (1991) 'The influence of education and social class on the diagnosis of dementia in a community population.' *Psychological Medicine 21*, 219–224.

Opit, L. and Pahl, J. (1993) 'Institutional care for elderly people: can we predict admissions?' *Research, Policy and Planning 10*, 2–5.

Orbell, S., Hopkins, N. and Gillies, B. (1993) 'Measuring the impact of informal caring.' *Journal of Community and Applied Social Psychology 3*, 149–163.

Parker, G. (1990) *With Due Care and Attention: A Review of Research on Informal Care.* (2nd edition) London: Family Policy Studies Centre.

Philp, I. and Young, J. (1988) 'An audit of a primary care team's knowledge of the existence of symptomatic demented elderly.' *Health Bulletin 46*, 93–97.

Philp, I. et al (1997) 'Factors associated with the maintenance and care of the demented elderly in the community.' *Ageing and Mental Health,* in press.

Philp, I., McKee, K.J., Meldrum, P., Ballinger, B.R., Gilhooly, M.L.M., Gordon, D.S., Mutch, W.J. and Whittick, J.E. (1995) 'Community care for demented and non-demented elderly people: a comparison study of financial burden, service use, and unmet needs in family supporters.' *British Medical Journal 310*, 1503–1506.

Preston, G.A.N. (1986) 'Dementia in elderly adults: prevalence and institutionalisation.' *Journal of Gerontology 41*, 261–267.

Primrose, W.R. and Capewell, A.E. (1986) 'A survey of registered nursing homes in Edinburgh.' *Journal of the Royal College of Physicians 36*, 125-128.

Schneider, J., Kavanagh, S., Knapp, M., Neechman, J. and Netten, A. (1993) 'Elderly people with advanced cognitive impairment in England: resource use and costs.' *Ageing and Society 13*, 27–50.

Schulz, R., Visintainer, P. and Williamson, G.M. (1990) 'Psychiatric and physical morbidity effects of caregiving.' *Journal of Gerontology 45*, P181–P191.

Scottish Office (1995) *Community Care Bulletin 1994.* Edinburgh: Statistical Bulletin Social Work Series SWK/CMC/1995/5.

Shah, A., Phongsathorn, V., George, C., Bielawska, C. and Katona, C. (1992) 'Psychiatric morbidity among continuing care geriatric inpatients.' *International Journal of Geriatric Psychiatry 7*, 517–525.

Shah, A., Phongsathorn, V., George, C., Bielawska, C. and Katona, C. (1993) 'Does psychiatric morbidity predict mortality in continuing care geriatric inpatients?' *International Journal of Geriatric Psychiatry 8*, 255–259.

Sinclair, I., Parker, R., Leat, D. and Williams, J. (1990) *The Kaleidoscope of Care: A Review of Research on Welfare Provision for Elderly People.* London: HMSO.

Spicker, P., Gordon, D.S., Ballinger, B.R., Mutch, W.J. and Seed, P. (1995) *Needs Assessment Package for Local Dementia Planning.* Scottish Office Home and Health Department Chief Scientist Office research grant K/OPR/2/2/C978.

Taylor, R., Ford, G. and Dunbar, M. (1995) 'The effects of caring on health: a community-based longitudinal study.' *Social Science and Medicine 40*, 1407–1415.

Wenger, G.C. (1990) 'Elderly carers: the need for appropriate intervention.' *Ageing and Society 10*, 197–219.

Wenger, G.C. (1994) 'Dementia sufferers living at home.' *International Journal of Geriatric Psychiatry 9*, 721–733.

Whalley, L.J., Thomas, B.M., McGonigal, G., McQuade, C., Swingler, R. and Black, R. (1995) 'Epidemiology of presenile Alzheimer's Disease in Scotland: non-random variation.' *British Journal of Psychiatry 167*, 728–731.

Wilkin, D. and Thompson, C. (1989) *Users' Guide to Dependency Measures for Elderly People.* Sheffield: University of Sheffield.

Williams, E.I., Savage, S., McDonald, P. and Groom, L. (1992) 'Residents of private nursing homes and their care.' *British Journal of General Practice 42*, 477–481.

Further reading

Blessed, G., Edwardson, J.A. and Kay, D.W.K. (1990) 'Prevalence rates of dementia in an ageing population: are low rates due to the use of insensitive instruments?' *Age and Ageing 19*, 84–90.

Brooks, P.W. (1992) 'Planning services for dementia.' *Health Bulletin 50*, 206–215.

Jorm, A., Henderson, A., Kay, D. and Jacomb, P. (1991) 'Mortality in relation to dementia, depression and social integration in an elderly community sample.' *International Journal of Geriatric Psychiatry 6*, 5–11.

Livingstone, G., Hawkins, A., Graham, N., Blizard, B. and Mann, A. (1990) 'The Gospel Oak study: prevalence rates of dementia, depression and activity limitation among elderly residents in Inner London.' *Psychological Medicine 20*, 137–146.

PART II
Selected Aspects of Dementia

Chapter 4

Early Onset Dementia

Lawrence Whalley

Introduction

Dementia describes the loss of mental faculties in adulthood. Decline in memory is a core feature of dementia, although reasoning and planning are also impaired. There are often changes in temperament and judgement but these are not essential for diagnosis. Mental impairment contrasts with mental disability which affects an individual's functioning at a personal level, often in everyday activities of daily living. These are also impaired in dementia, such that deficits arise in self-care as a consequence of mental impairment. In a much wider social context, individuals with dementia are not only disabled but are also handicapped, such that their social functioning is hindered as a direct consequence of mental impairment. Both the disabilities and handicaps can, in turn, be much modified by the social context within which a dementia sufferer is expected to function.

Dementia incidence increases rapidly with age (Jorm 1990). At about 40 years of age, fewer than 1 per 1000 of the at risk population have been admitted to hospital for investigation of dementia. By this age, perhaps 3 or 4 more per 1000 have also developed cognitive impairment but have not been admitted to hospital. Somewhat more men than women are affected by dementia before age 65, when about 50 per 1000 of the at risk population have been admitted to hospital because of dementia. The steady exponential rise between ages 40 and 64 continues into old age, doubling at approximately five-yearly intervals until age about 90 years, when there is some evidence of a levelling out or even a fall (Jorm *et al.* 1987). Women outnumber men in these older age groups for reasons other than their greater longevity. Older textbooks of psychiatry use the terms 'presenium' and 'senile' to an extent that the term 'disease' was used to describe dementias arising before age 65, and the term 'senile dementia' described a group of disorders widely believed to be a consequence of the inevitable neuro-degeneration of ageing. The terms 'presenile' and 'senile' are now archaic; early onset and late onset are preferred.

The onset of dementia in an individual of working age who may have extensive family responsibilities (to spouse, children and, possibly, parents) is often viewed as a personal tragedy. Especially in the initial stages of early onset dementia, sufferers remain at least partially insightful into the nature of their impairments. Depression, anxiety and, sometimes, paranoid feelings are not unusual. Relatives, likewise, begin to feel the loss of the person they knew. Plans for holidays, retirement and joint ventures are laid aside as the burden of care increases and, for a spouse, sole responsibility is assumed for family, financial and social affairs.

Current research suggests that the terms 'early onset' and 'late onset' dementia possess particular causal and management implications (Breitner 1991: Breitner *et al.* 1988). Molecular genetic techniques have succeeded in the identification of specific genetic factors that act most often in early onset patients. Because these factors are genetically determined but have not become apparent until middle age, their recognition may distress the children of the recent onset dementia patient. The social and psychological consequences of an early onset dementia of this type are probably much more extensive within the family than is the case with late onset dementia.

The identification of specific genetic factors in early onset dementia has been the greatest benefit obtained from the past 15 years of research in clinical neurobiology. No other group of major mental illnesses or impairments has been elucidated so thoroughly. In turn, this success has raised public expectations of the treatment of these devastating illnesses, much as the cinema has altered public perceptions of autism and the adreno-leukodystrophies with films such as *Rain Man* and *Lorenzo's Oil*. The pessimistic view that the dementias of middle age are unfortunate accidents of the ageing process and should be regarded with much pessimism and therapeutic indifference no longer sits comfortably with increased public awareness of the substantial advances in clinical neuroscience. Research workers have responded by promoting a climate of informed circumspection in this regard. Scientific meetings on dementia rarely pass without organised discussion of the social and ethical issues involved and their implications for the individual, the family and society. In broad terms, these issues concern the use of molecular genetic techniques in pre-symptomatic diagnosis; the estimation of genetic risk; the use of experimental treatments in individuals who cannot, because of dementia, give their 'informed consent'; the possibility that anti-dementia treatments may, initially, be only of partial effect and so succeed in slowing the progress of a dementia and thereby prolonging the suffering of the patient; the use of implanted nerve cells taken from healthy aborted foetuses; and, lastly, the health-economic consequences of the availability of effective anti-dementia treatment that may be both expensive to administer and serve to prolong the dependency of the affected individual on state support.

The causes of early onset dementia

Alzheimer's disease

Alzheimer's disease is a degenerative disorder of the brain. It is chronic and progressive and, inevitably, leads to death, usually within about seven years of symptom onset (Lishman 1987). A definitive diagnosis is possible only after death. Individuals with early onset Alzheimer's disease are more likely to have a family history of dementia, usually of Alzheimer's disease (Breitner et al. 1988). Patients with Down's syndrome are at a high risk of developing Alzheimer's disease in middle age, as described by Holland in Chapter 6 of this volume. A broad range of clinical features is encountered in early onset Alzheimer's disease. There are two main groups of symptoms, labelled 'cognitive' and 'behavioural', although they should not be seen as independent. Cognitive symptoms include deficits in memory, intellect and reasoning with associated disturbances in consciousness and attention. Behavioural symptoms include hallucinations and delusions, disturbance in mood and symptoms such as wandering. Environmental factors in early onset Alzheimer's disease may be of particular relevance, especially in light of recent support for the, 'low educational attainment hypothesis of Alzheimer's disease' (Mortimer 1995). Most factors have been the subject of considerable controversy, largely because of the lack of statistical power found in each study. This was overcome by a meta-analysis of high quality case control studies of environmental factors in Alzheimer's disease (van Duijn et al. 1991). More recently, population-based studies have supported low educational attainment as a predisposing factor for Alzheimer's disease (Mortimer and Graves 1993). Generally speaking, less well-educated people perform less well on mental status tests in old age. At first, the possible association between low education and dementia was thought to be artifactual, but as studies became more sophisticated so the link became better established (Mortimer 1995). Current explanations of the putative link between low education and an increased risk of dementia include:

1. Low socio-economic status and education are associated in adult life with increased exposure to occupational neurotoxins or environmental hazards that could harm brain cells.

2. Low educational attainment is associated with low socio-economic status at birth and, in turn, involved with diminished access to good nutrition and health care. In such circumstances, neurodevelopmental insults might be more likely or less well repaired and this, in turn, could predispose to dementia in late life.

3. Conversely, high educational attainment might lead to a more active brain which develops a richness in communication between brain cells and facility of use that mitigates the effects of the dementing process and is not available to others of low education.

Cerebrovascular disease and early onset dementia

Cerebrovascular disease is an important risk factor for early onset dementia (Haschinski 1992). Most often seen in the dementia that follows stroke where an acute episode of disturbed consciousness is followed by confusion and signs of nervous system damage; cognitive impairment is detectable in about 25 per cent of those who survive the acute episode. The risk factors for vascular dementia include increasing age, a history of stroke, low education, hypertension, a history of myocardial infarction, diabetes and a history of 'falls' (Breteler *et al.* 1994). The assessment of patients with features suggestive of vascular dementia must include a detailed medical examination. The risk factors for vascular dementia (and its progression) are potentially reversible and merit high quality clinical care.

Other causes of early onset dementia
DEMENTIA ASSOCIATED WITH PARKINSON'S DISEASE

About 30 per cent of old people progress to dementia. There are no good estimates of the development of cognitive impairment in early onset Parkinson's disease, but these seem likely to be similar to those found in older people. Almost always, the signs and symptoms of Parkinson's disease begin some years before the onset of the dementing illness. Typical dementia features in Parkinson's disease include poor concentration, indecisiveness and difficulty in maintaining attention and motivation. Whereas the Parkinsonian features respond to dopaninergic drug therapies, there is little evidence that the cognitive features will do likewise.

HUMAN IMMUNO DEFICIENCY VIRUS (HIV) AND EARLY ONSET DEMENTIA

There are numerous neurological complications of the Acquired Immuno Deficiency Syndrome (AIDS). In addition to opportunistic infection of the nervous system, the HIV virus causes disease of brain cells. Initially, the AIDS dementia complex proved very difficult to describe and did not gain immediate acceptance. In large part, this was attributable to the complexity of the relationship between the neuropathological changes in HIV and the clinical symptoms of dementia. Not surprisingly, AIDS patients may suffer multiple reasons for cognitive impairment other than the direct action of the HIV virus. These include the psychotoxic effects of AIDS treatment, the effects on brain functioning of intercurrent infections, the debilitating effects of long-term illness, and psychological reactions to the terminal phase of illness. These facts make estimations of the number of AIDS patients who suffer 'early onset dementia' very difficult indeed. In terms of patient management, the problem of 'AIDS dementia' does not figure greatly within the context it is encountered. Such patients have so many other life-threatening illnesses and related matters to contend with that their cognitive impairment does not attract much therapeutic interest.

HUNTINGTON'S DISEASE

Huntington's disease is a rare genetic cause of early onset dementia. The association between semi-purposeful dance-like (choreiform) movements and dementia prompted the term 'Huntington's Chorea' which is now obsolete. Typically, there are about 6 or 7 cases of Huntington's Chorea per 100,000 at risk. The onset of the disease is usually between ages 25 and 50, with an average in the mid-40s. Importantly, a family history, although present, is not infrequently unavailable and the diagnosis in an adult or middle-aged individual can be quite unexpected by the patient and family. Consequently, the patient's siblings and children may become aware of the risk that they might also succumb to the condition. Seen in these terms, the observed low incidence of Huntington's disease is a substantial underestimate of the public health problem posed by the condition. For every affected Huntington's patient there will be others who are unaffected but have not yet completed the period of risk, some of whom may at the time of diagnosis in a parent, be considering marriage and the prospect of raising a family of their own. These effects of Huntington's disease are compounded by the relatively long survival from disease onset to death which is, typically, about 15 to 20 years.

PICK'S DISEASE AND FRONTAL LOBE DEMENTIA

Pick's disease and the frontal lobe dementias are among the least frequently encountered causes of early onset dementia. The most distinctive clinical features are of characteristic social and behavioural changes rather than the impairments of memory and reasoning that so characterise the other types of early onset dementia.

SPONGIFORM ENCEPHALOPATHIES

This is a rare group of diseases first described by Creutzfeldt and Jakob (Creutzfeldt-Jakob disease; CJD). There is currently considerable public, professional and press interest in the incidence of these spongiform encephalopyosis and this may, in turn, have served to improve the detection of cases. There are about 50 to 70 new cases of human spongiform encephalopathy in the United Kingdom every year. From onset to death is generally less than one year and there are diverse neurological and psychiatric symptoms and signs. Clinical descriptions of presentation and course of the illness have been so varied that without neuropathological validation and in the absence of a valid laboratory diagnostic test, it is generally thought hazardous to make the diagnosis. Occasionally cerebral biopsy in life is justified to obtain such confirma'.ion.

A family history of a similar dementia is present in about one in seven cases of spongiform encephalopathy.

ALCOHOLIC DEMENTIA

Popular perceptions of alcoholism include the notion that a substantial proportion of those who have become physically dependent upon alcohol for ten or more years will certainly have suffered some form of 'brain damage'. No consensus exists concerning the term 'alcoholic dementia' which has been applied variously to: (1) those alcoholics who show persistent characteristic cognitive deficits in the face of prolonged abstinence (Korsakoff's psychosis); (2) alcoholic individuals from socio-economically disadvantaged backgrounds who have a history of alcohol dependence, head trauma, poor nutritional status and poor health, but who are rarely abstinent for a sufficient period to determine if the cognitive impairments persist in the absence of alcohol; and (3) alcoholic individuals of previously low educational attainment and a history of recidivism and institutionalisation who also perform badly on neuropsychological testing. Unfortunately, precise definitions of these (and related) variants do not perform well in population-based studies and data are unavailable to determine precisely the size of the problem of alcoholic dementia in the community. The general principle applies that those alcoholics who have least social support and whose drinking pattern is associated with rapid rises in blood alcohol are more likely to cause public and legal concern, whereas those alcoholics who are better able to use health services are most often identified in community surveys.

Neuropsychological studies show that, when abstinent, those who have been dependent upon alcohol perform less well on tests of psychomotor speed, perceptional motor functioning, visuo-spatial competence, measures of abstracting ability and complex reasoning, even after 12 months' total abstinence. These deficits are usually of a mild to moderate degree and it is contentious if they interfere with independent functioning to a noticeable degree. In large part, this accounts for the reluctance to accept the concept of 'alcoholic dementia'. In addition, there is also the emerging view that some of these deficits are partially reversible after prolonged abstinence and nutritional enrichment. The term 'reversible alcoholic dementia' is sometimes used but has not gained wide acceptance.

The validity of 'alcoholic dementia' would be strengthened if direct neuropathological evidence could be presented in support. Unfortunately, this is not the case. Wernicke's encephalopathy and Korsakoff's psychosis have distinct neuropathological changes but are relatively rare causes of cognitive impairment in alcoholics. The majority who show persistent cognitive deficit have only minimal structural changes in the brain and these are difficult to detect in neuro-imaging studies. The likelihood of better based community studies of alcohol-dependent individuals with careful neuropsychological and brain imaging measurements should go some way towards resolving the nature and extent of the problem posed by the 'alcoholic dementias'.

In conclusion most believe effective therapies, whilst feasible, are decades away, yet acknowledge that the benefits of any new treatment will not be detected until important clinical and socio-ethical issues have been effectively addressed. Meanwhile, only about 50 per cent of people identified by hospitals and clinics as having early onset dementia remain in touch with services two years later. This points to the importance of early onset dementia sufferers being offered a package of caring services designed to promote high medical standards of investigation, diagnosis and clinical management that is closely integrated with community-based supporting services.

References

Breitner, J.C.S. (1991) 'Clinical genetics and genetic counselling in Alzheimer's disease.' *Ann. Int. Med. 115*, 601–606.

Breitner, J.C.S., Silverman, J.M., Mohs, R.C. extd. (1988) 'Familial aggregation in Alzheimer's disease: comparison of risk among relatives of early onset and late onset cases and among male and female relatives in successive generations.' *Neurology 38*, 207–212.

Breteler, M.M., van Sweiten, J.C., Bots, M. *et al.* (1994) 'Cerebral white matter lesions, vascular risk factors and cognitive function in a population-based study: the Rotterdam Study.' *Neurology 44*, 1246–1252.

Haschinski, V. (1992) 'Preventable senility: a call for action against vascular dementias.' *Lancet 340*, 645–648.

Jorm, A.F. (1990) *The Epidemiology of Alzheimer's Disease and Related Disorders.* London: Chapman and Hall.

Jorm, A.F., Korten, A.E. and Henderson, A.S. (1987) 'The prevalence of dementia: a quantitative integration of the literature.' *Acta Psychiat. Scan. 76*, 456–479.

Lishman, W.A. (1987) *Organic Psychiatry* (second edition). Oxford: Blackwell Science.

Mortimer, J.A. (1995) 'The epidemiology of Alzheimer's disease: beyond risk factors in research advances in Alzheimer's disease and related disorders.' In K. Igbal, J. Mortimer, B. Winblad and H.M. Wisnieswk (eds) (J. Wiley).

Mortimer, J. and Graves, A. (1993) 'Education and other socioeconomic determinants of dementia and Alzheimer's disease.' *Neurology 43* (Suppl. 4), 539–544.

van Duijn, C.M., de Kniff, P., Cruts, M. *et al.* (1991) 'Apilipoprokin E 4 allele in a population-based study of early-onset Alzheimer's disease.' *Nature Genet. 7*, 74–78.

Chapter 5

Depression and Dementia

Jill Warrington

Depression in older people

Defining depression

Depression in elderly people is an important cause of increased morbidity and mortality (Murphy 1983; Murphy *et al.* 1988) and presents particular diagnostic challenges. The term 'depression' is used clinically to apply to a spectrum of disorders which are classified and described in the *Diagnostic and Statistical Manual of Mental Disorders 4th Edition* (American Psychiatric Association 1994). Broadly speaking, three main disorders are described: major depressive episode, dysthymia and adjustment disorder. The first of these can be thought of as the most severe form of depression and is likely to include symptoms such as depressed, disinterested or irritable mood associated with loss of interest or pleasure in activities. In addition, the capacity for enjoyment is diminished, with difficulty in concentrating, lethargy, sleep and appetite disturbance, and decreased self-esteem and self-confidence. Ideas of guilt, worthlessness or suicide may occur.

Dysthymia is a lower grade but chronic disturbance of mood on most days which lasts for over two years. Adjustment disorders are milder and relatively short-lived disturbances of mood, appearing within three months of a stressor and causing significant distress and impaired functioning.

In older people the presenting complaint is more likely to be of anxiety, bodily symptoms or memory problems than of low mood (Meyers and Alexopoulos 1988).

Epidemiology

Estimates of the prevalence of depression in older people vary widely. There are considerable difficulties in carrying out epidemiological studies, and results vary depending on the population studied and the criteria adopted in defining depression.

In community-based studies using interview schedules specifically designed for older people, an average of approximately 15 per cent of subjects have significant depressive illness. These people would be considered to require treatment in routine clinical practice. The number fulfilling the criteria for DSM IV (American Psychiatric Association 1994) major depression is reported to be much smaller at 1–5 per cent (Blazer 1994).

In institutional settings, most studies report higher rates of depression than in the community. Generally these studies include only those residents who are able to complete the interview and may therefore exclude people with dementia who may also be depressed. Studies of prevalence of significant depression among residents of residential care homes would suggest that 20–40 per cent may be significantly depressed (Harrison, Sawa and Kafetz 1990; Macdonald and Dunn 1982; Mann, Graham and Ashby 1984; Phillips and Henderson 1991).

Aetiology

Understanding the factors which contribute to the development and maintenance of depression in elderly people is important for several reasons. It is helpful in explaining the high prevalence of significant depression in elderly people, in identifying those who may be most at risk and in developing management strategies which will relieve symptoms.

Neurochemical theories of depression are well described and have informed the development of antidepressant drug treatment as well as helping to explain why many drugs cause depression. Genetics play a part, but less so in those elderly people who develop a depressive illness for the first time in old age (Alexopoulos 1989). Psychological theories, including the behavioural, cognitive and psychoanalytical, are of great importance and the underlying principles are of particular significance to those providing services for older people. Psychosocial factors such as the lack of a confiding relationship and life events such as bereavement increase the risk of depression in some older people (Murphy 1982). Physical illness, including parkinsonism, carcinoma or cardiovascular disease, is another significant risk factor.

A combination of biological, psychological and social factors may interact in predisposing an individual to depression or in precipitating or maintaining that depression. The high prevalence of some of the biological (e.g. physical illness) and social (e.g. bereavement) risk factors in the older population may be further increased in those requiring residential care.

Recognition

The symptoms described above are the basis on which depression should be recognised. In addition, an appreciation of the aetiological factors and a high index of suspicion, given the prevalence rates, are invaluable. There is evidence that detection rates are low, both in the community by general practitioners (Iliffe *et al.* 1991) and in nursing homes by physicians and nursing staff (Rovner *et al.* 1991). As a consequence, depressive symptoms in these circumstances are untreated (Rovner *et al.* 1991).

The relationship between depression and dementia

Depression and dementia have a close but complex relationship, the understanding of which remains the subject of investigation. Both conditions exist along continua which appear to intersect at various points of clinical significance (Emery and Oxman 1992). Depression may exist with or without clinically significant cognitive deficit. In a small number of cases, the deficit may be sufficiently severe to present as dementia. This condition is referred to as 'depressive dementia' or 'pseudodementia' and will be discussed in more detail below. Similarly, dementia may occur with or without clinically meaningful depressive symptoms. Where depression occurs it may be as a secondary condition to dementia or as an independent condition, often in people who have suffered recurrent depression prior to developing dementia.

The relationship between depression and dementia is further complicated by the presence of shared symptoms and the effects of either depressed mood or cognitive impairment on the ability to express those symptoms.

Depressive dementia (pseudodementia)

The terms 'depressive dementia' or 'pseudodementia' are not diagnostic terms but serve as a reminder that some severely depressed patients may present as if they have dementia and perform poorly on memory tests. It is likely that approximately 10 per cent of people given an initial diagnosis of dementia will have a treatable cause for their symptoms. The most common treatable cause is depression (McLean 1987). In depressive dementia the most prominent symptom is often the inability to think or concentrate, which may lead to complaints of poor memory. Table 5.1 gives an indication of features which help distinguish depressive dementia from organic dementia. Many of these features were originally described by Wells (1979) and are generally supported (Feinberg and Goodman 1984).

**Table 5.1: Distinguishing features between
depressive dementia and dementia**

	Depressive dementia	Dementia
History	Onset gradual but may be dated accurately	Onset insidious and vague
	Symptoms progress rapidly over weeks or months	Symptoms progress slowly over months or years
	Previous or family history of depression common	Previous or family history of depression less likely
	Family very aware of disability early on	Family usually unaware of disability until later
	Early morning wakening may occur	Nocturnal wandering and confusion
	Patient complains of memory loss	Patient rarely complains of memory loss
	Patient emphasises the disability	Patient hides the disability
	Symptoms often worse in the morning	Disorientation may be worse in the evening
Examination	Patient is distressed	Mood is unpredictably labile
	Observed mood is altered from normal	Overall change in mood is not observed
	Thoughts are sad and hopeless and may be slowed	Thoughts tend to be repetitive, slow andreflect reduced interest
	Tend to give 'don't know' answers to questions	Give incorrect answers
	Performance in testing is variable	Performance is consistently poor
	Gaps in memory are apparent	Memory loss is more global – specific gaps are rare

Table 5.1: Distinguishing features between depressive dementia and dementia (continued)

Depressive dementia	*Dementia*
Remote memory is intact	Remote memory may be impaired
Little effort is made in answering	Patients tend to try hard to answer questions
Cortical functionsare spared – seldom aphasia, apraxia, agnosia	Usually impaired cortical functions
Mood congruent auditory hallucinations in 20% of sufferers	Hallucinations if present often visual

All those involved in the care of elderly people have a role to play in gathering information which allows such a diagnosis to be made. In some cases, a trial of antidepressant treatment is required to clarify the diagnosis.

In the short term, the prognosis for people with depressive dementia who receive adequate treatment is good. Most will recover following treatment with antidepressant drugs. In very severe cases, particularly where symptoms do not respond to drug treatment, electro-convulsive therapy may be indicated. The importance of good psychosocial support while treatment is ongoing cannot be overemphasised. In the longer term, however, it would appear that the majority of these patients go on to develop dementia if followed up for a lengthy period. As many as 89 per cent developed dementia when followed for eight years in one study (Kral and Emery 1989).

Depression in older people with an established diagnosis of dementia

As described above, depression can occur as a secondary condition in people with dementia or as an ongoing pattern of recurrent depressive episodes which pre-date the onset of dementia.

Epidemiology

Wide variations are reported in the prevalence of depressive symptoms and depressive syndromes in the literature. The mean prevalence of depressive symptoms in Alzheimer's disease is likely to be around 30 per cent for symptoms and 20 per cent for syndromes. Major depressive episodes are relatively rare (Allen and Burns 1995). Depression may be more common in people with Lewy body dementia or multi-infarct dementia (McKeith et al. 1992; Sultzer et al. 1993).

Aetiology

The aetiological factors applicable to depression also apply in depression co-existing with dementia.

Biological factors may be of particular significance, as the destruction of particular areas of the brain and neurochemical pathways leads to increased incidence of depression. Neurochemically the brains of people diagnosed to be suffering both depression and dementia show lower levels of noradrenalin in the cortex than those who suffered dementia alone (Zubenko, Moossy and Kopp 1990). Left frontal brain damage in stroke is associated with depression (Starkstein and Robinson 1989). Depression occurs at all stages of dementia but seems to be more common in the earlier stages (Burns, Jacoby and Levy 1990). This has led to suggestions that the extreme alteration of brain functioning may be protective in the later stages of dementia or that psychological factors become less important as dementia progresses.

The possible psychological mechanisms which may help in explaining why depression exists so commonly with dementia have not been well explored. In some cases, depression may be an understandable reaction to the losses of dementia. Insight into these losses is less likely to be present as the dementia progresses (Feher *et al.* 1991). Although this may help explain the finding that depression is more common in the earlier stages of dementia, two studies have failed to find an association between the presence of insight and depressive symptoms (Feher *et al.* 1991; Verhey *et al.* 1993).

The importance of depression as a response to life events in people with dementia has also been addressed. Relocation can be detrimental and may lead to depressive behaviour in people with dementia (Anthony *et al.* 1987). People with dementia are just as susceptible to the development of depression in response to life events as those who are cognitively intact. Change in routine has a role, but this is likely to be secondary to a strong association between severe threat and depression in people with dementia (Orrell and Bebbington 1995).

Recognition

The challenge of identifying which people with dementia are also suffering significant depression is made greater by the shared symptomatology of the two conditions. Loss of motivation, decreased energy, agitation or retardation, altered sleep and appetite can be features of either condition. Gathering detailed information about the onset and nature of these symptoms is essential and involves all team members. Listening to carers and staff members who note a change in the person with dementia which is 'not his normal dementia' is crucial. Of particular importance are changes in sleep pattern, appetite and level of arousal.

In very early dementia, the symptoms and signs of depression are no different from those experienced by people who do not have dementia. People with dementia, including those with mild dementia, under-report their depressive symptoms (Teri and Wagner 1991). They may not complain consistently and are reported to be particularly able to be 'cheered up' (Merriam *et al.* 1988). In later stages, the distress associated with depression may be demonstrated through behaviour change and problems including incontinence, agitation, suspiciousness, restlessness and aggression (Teri and Wagner 1992). The finding that people with co-existing depression and dementia show additional impairment of instrumental activities of daily living is also significant (Pearson *et al.* 1989). This additional disability, in terms of behavioural disturbance and impaired self-care, is particularly important in those individuals developing depression at an early stage of dementia where abilities might otherwise be preserved.

The changes in behaviour associated with depression appear to be particularly difficult for carers of people with dementia. Carers report high levels of strain, burden and distress in association with withdrawn behaviour, emotional distress and other depression-related behaviours in the person with dementia (Greene *et al.* 1982; Teri and Wagner 1992).

Given that the presenting problems associated with depression in dementia are so variable and may also reflect deterioration in the dementia, staff need further guidance in recognising the symptoms of depression in people with dementia. Awareness of how a person makes staff members feel (e.g. sad or hopeless) can be an important clue. Listening to the person with dementia, however disjointed their speech, may reveal themes of fear, gloom or hopelessness which can indicate depression.

Management of depression in people with dementia
There is no place for therapeutic nihilism in the treatment of people with co-existing depression and dementia. Effective treatments are available, although most merit further investigation.

A culture of care which embraces principles of personhood, thereby preserving self-esteem and a feeling of worth, is a good starting point in the management of depression in people with dementia (Kitwood 1993). Addressing the quality of the social environment has a positive effect on mood (Minde, Haynes and Rodenburgh 1990). Dementia care mapping may prove useful in improving the quality of care interactions and may have an effect on depression (Kitwood and Bredin 1992).

Behavioural theories of depression are particularly relevant to people with dementia. Apathy, lack of initiative and loss of skills lead to withdrawal from activity. The loss of pleasurable activity results in depressed mood with further withdrawal and deepening depression (Lewinsohn, Seeley and Fischer 1991). Staff must be aware of their role in initiating and maintaining pleasurable activities of any type for people with dementia. Formal psychological therapies, both individual and group, have also been used with people with dementia (Bonder 1994). As yet no clinical trials of their effectiveness in treating depression in this group have been reported.

Antidepressant drug treatment has not been thoroughly evaluated in the treatment of depression co-existing with dementia. Clinical impressions, controlled and uncontrolled trials suggest it is effective (Reifler *et al.* 1989). Newer drugs, such as the modified tricyclics, the selective serotonin reuptake inhibitors and noradrenalin reuptake inhibitors, have fewer side effects and are less likely to be fatal if taken in overdose. Antidepressants must be prescribed in suitable dosage for an adequate period of time and may require to be continued in order to prevent relapse.

It is important that treatment is not denied, because depressive symptoms are understandable. Understanding is important in that it promotes empathy, but where significant depressive symptoms, which represent a change from the person's norm, are present, treatment should be considered. Similarly whether or not depression is understandable should not dictate the type of treatment offered. Where simple behavioural measures fail to produce resolution, both physical and psychological treatment should be considered. Drug treatment often has a place in resolving distressing symptoms and allowing the person to participate more effectively in other aspects of treatment.

Implications for services

Given that depression co-existing with dementia is common, leads to increased care needs and is treatable, there are likely to be considerable benefits in improving recognition and treatment.

Communication within services is vital and can be improved by minimising staff turnover and encouraging comprehensive handover of information between staff groups. This ensures changes are noted and clients feel able to confide when necessary. Attention must be paid to effective liaison between all members of the multidisciplinary team and, in particular, contact with mental health professionals should be encouraged. Managers must ensure treatment recommendations are clearly understood by all staff and are followed through. The implementation of suggested interventions (psychiatric, social and medical) has been found to be lacking, perhaps due to lack of resources and poor co-operation between disciplines (Ames 1990). Such deficiencies should be noted and audit processes applied to improve practice. Exposure to successful treatment will both educate and encourage staff.

Many of the measures which are likely to benefit people with co-existing depression and dementia, such as the standard of the environment, appropriate enjoyable activities and the opportunity to speak with, and be heard by, professional care-givers, should form the basis of quality care in all settings. In addition, effective treatment for depression is available and encouraging staff to make careful observations should ensure it is requested and delivered.

References

Alexopoulos, G.S. (1989) 'Biological abnormalities in late life depression.' *Journal of Geriatric Psychiatry 141,* 25–34.

Allen, H.N.P. and Burns, A. (1995) 'The non-cognitive features of dementia.' *Reviews of Clinical Gerontology 5,* 57–78.

American Psychiatric Association (1994) *Diagnostic and Statistical Manual of Mental Disorders 4th Edition.* Washington, DC: American Psychiatric Association.

Ames, D. (1990) 'Depression among elderly residents of local authority residential homes – its nature and the efficacy of intervention.' *British Journal of Psychiatry 156,* 667–675.

Anthony, V., Procter, A.W., Silverman, A.M. and Murphy, E. (1987) 'Mood and behaviour problems following the relocation of elderly patients with mental illness.' *Age and Ageing 16,* 355–365.

Blazer, D.G. (1994) 'Epidemiology of depression: prevalence and incidence.' In J.M.R. Copeland, M.T. Abou-Saleh and D.G. Blazer (eds) *Principles and Practice of Geriatric Psychiatry.* Chichester: John Wiley and Sons.

Bonder, B.R. (1994) 'Psychotherapy for individuals with Alzheimer's disease.' *Alzheimer's Disease and Associated Disorders 8* (Suppl. 3), 75–81.

Burns, A., Jacoby, R. and Levy, R. (1990) 'Psychiatric phenomena in Alzheimer's disease: 3. Disorders of mood.' *British Journal of Psychiatry 157,* 81–86.

Emery, V.O. and Oxman, T.E. (1992) 'Update on the dementia spectrum of depression.' *American Journal of Psychiatry 149*, 305–317.

Feher, E.P., Mahurin, R.K., Inbody, S.B., Crook, T.H. and Pirozzolo, F.J. (1991) 'Anosognosia in Alzheimer's disease.' *Neuropsychiatry, Neuropsychology and Behavioural Neurology 4*, 136–146.

Feinberg, T. and Goodman, B. (1984) 'Affective illness, dementia and pseudodementia.' *Journal of Clinical Psychiatry 45*, 99–103.

Greene, J.G., Smith, B., Gardiner, M. and Timbury, G.C. (1982) 'Measuring behavioural disturbance of elderly demented patients in the community and its effects on relatives: a factor analytic study.' *Age and Ageing 11*, 121–126.

Harrison, R., Sawa, N. and Kafetz, K. (1990) 'Dementia depression and physical disability in a London borough: a survey of elderly people in and out of residential care and implications for future developments.' *Age and Ageing 19*, 97–103.

Iliffe, S., Haines, A., Gallivan, S. Booroff, A., Gottenberg, E. and Morgan, P. (1991) 'Assessment of elderly people in general practice 1. Social circumstances and mental state.' *British Journal of General Practice 41*, 9–12.

Kitwood, T. (1993) 'Person and process in dementia.' *International Journal of Geriatric Psychiatry 8*, 541–545.

Kitwood, T. and Bredin, K. (1992) 'A new approach to the evaluation of dementia care.' *Journal of Advances in Health and Nursing Care 1*, 5, 41–60.

Kral, V.A. and Emery, O.B. (1989) 'Long term follow up of depressive pseudodementia of the aged.' *Canadian Journal of Psychiatry 34*, 445–446.

Lewinsohn, P.R., Seeley, J.R. and Fischer, S.A. (1991) 'Age and depression: unique and shared effects.' *Psychology and Ageing 6*, 247–260.

Macdonald, A.J.D. and Dunn, J. (1982) 'Death and the expressed wish to die in the elderly: an outcome study.' *Age and Ageing 11*, 189–195.

Mann, A.H., Graham, N. and Ashby, D. (1984) 'Psychiatric illness in residential homes for the elderly: a survey in one London borough.' *Age and Ageing 13*, 257–265.

McKeith, I.G., Perry, R.H., Fairburn, A.F., Jabeen, S. and Perry, E.K. (1992) 'Operational criteria for senile dementia of Lewy body type (SDLT).' *Psychological Medicine 22*, 911–922.

McLean, S. (1987) 'Assessing dementia, Part 1: difficulties, definitions and clinical diagnosis.' *Australia and New Zealand Journal of Psychiatry 21*, 142–174.

Merriam, A.E., Aronson, M.K., Gaston, P., Wey, S.L. and Katz, I. (1988) 'The psychiatric symptoms of Alzheimer's disease.' *Journal of the American Geriatrics Society 36*, 7–12.

Meyers, B.S. and Alexopoulos, G.S. (1988) 'Geriatric depression.' *Medical Clinics of North America 72*, 847–866.

Minde, R., Haynes, E. and Rodenburgh, M. (1990) 'The ward milieu and its effects on the behaviour of psychogeriatric patients.' *Canadian Journal of Psychiatry 35*, 133–138.

Murphy, E. (1982) 'Social origins of depression in old age.' *British Journal of Psychiatry 141*, 135–142.

Murphy, E. (1983) 'The prognosis of depression in old age.' *British Journal of Psychiatry 142*,111–119.

Murphy, E., Smith, R., Lindesay, L. and Slattery, J. (1988) 'Increased mortality in late life depression.' *British Journal of Psychiatry 152*, 347–353.

Orrell, M. and Bebbington, P. (1995) 'Life events and senile dementia 2: affective symptoms.' *British Journal of Psychiatry 166*, 613–620.

Pearson, J., Teri, L., Reifler, B. and Raskind, M. (1989) 'Functional status and cognitive impairment in Alzheimer's disease patients with and without depression.' *Journal of the American Geriatric Society 39*, 1117–1121.

Phillips, C.J. and Henderson, A.S. (1991) 'The prevalence of depression among Australian nursing home residents: results using draft ICD10 and DSMIIIR criteria.' *Psychological Medicine 21*, 739–748.

Reifler, B.V., Teri, L., Raskind, M., Veith, R., Barnes, R., White, E. and McLean, P. (1989) 'Double-blind trial of imipramine in Alzheimer's disease patients with and without depression.' *American Journal of Psychiatry 146*, 45–49.

Rovner, B.W., German, P.S., Brant, L.J., Clark, R., Burton, L. and Folstein, M.F. (1991) 'Depression and mortality in nursing homes.' *Journal of the American Medical Association 265*, 8, 993–996.

Starkstein, S.E. and Robinson, R.G. (1989) 'Affective disorders and cerebrovascular disease.' *British Journal of Psychiatry 154*, 170–182.

Sultzer, D.L., Levin, H.S., Mahler, M.E., High, W.M. and Cummings, J.L. (1993) 'A comparison of psychiatric symptoms in vascular dementia and Alzheimer's disease.' *American Journal of Psychiatry 150*, 1806–1812.

Teri, L. and Wagner, A. (1991) 'Assessment of depression in patients with Alzheimer's disease: concordance between informants.' *Psychology and Ageing 6*, 280–285.

Teri, L. and Wagner, A. (1992) 'Alzheimer's disease and depression.' *Journal of Consulting and Clinical Psychology 60*, 3, 379–391.

Verhey, F.R.J., Rozendaal, N., Ponds, R.W. and Jolles, J. (1993) 'Dementia awareness and depression.' *International Journal of Geriatric Psychiatry 8*, 851–856.

Wells, C.E. (1979) 'Pseudodementia.' *American Journal of Psychiatry 136*, 895–900.

Zubenko, G.S., Moosy, J. and Kopp, U. (1990) 'Neurochemical correlates of major depression in primary dementia.' *Archives Neurology 47*, 209–214.

Further reading

Post, F. and Shulman, K. (1985) 'New views on old age affective disorders.' In T. Airie (ed) *Recent Advances in Psychogeriatrics*, no.1. London: Churchill Livingstone.

Chapter 6

The Risk of Dementia in People with Down's Syndrome

Tony Holland

Introduction

There are several hundred genetic, chromosomal and environmentally determined causes of developmental delay in early childhood which result in significant intellectual impairment and the presence of learning disabilities. New genetic techniques are making possible the searching of the human genome and thereby the discovery of further chromosomal or single gene disorders (Flint *et al.* 1995). There has been strong criticism of what has been seen, certainly in the past, as an overemphasis on 'diagnostic labels', but as knowledge increases it has become apparent that specific causes of learning disabilities may result in an increased propensity to specific types of cognitive deficits, specific problem behaviours or particular physical or mental health problems. For this reason, knowing the cause of the developmental disability may have important consequences. In addition, this is essential if the family wishes for genetic advice and, furthermore, knowing the cause of a child's disability can be critical in aiding parents and other family members in their emotional adjustment.

Down's syndrome is a good illustration of these principles. Langdon Down first described the physical features characteristic of this particular syndrome in 1866 (see Berg (1993) for a summary). The cause was discovered by Lejeune *et al.* in 1959, three years after it had become possible to culture blood cells and visualise human chromosomes. The majority of people with DS were found to have three rather than the normal two copies of chromosome 21 (trisomy 21). Later, much rarer chromosomal variants resulting in partial trisomy 21 (translocations) or in only some cells having the extra copy (mosaicism) were reported (see the review by Hamerton 1982). These and other observations, together with the finding of a greater chance of the birth of a child with Down's syndrome with increased maternal age (Penrose 1939), have established the basis for the genetic advice given to the relatives of a child with Down's syndrome as well as informing UK prenatal screening policies.

Numerous studies have investigated the particular strengths and disabilities of children with Down's syndrome, including profiles of cognitive, emotional and language development and descriptions of the various physical problems, such as congenital heart disorders, gastrointestinal disorders and sensory impairments, which occur in excess (see Ciccheti and Beeghley 1990). A detailed study of a cohort of children born with Down's syndrome and followed into adult life has also illustrated the extent to which children and young adults with Down's syndrome can differ from each other and how the nature of their development changes over time (Carr 1995). In addition the establishment of the Down's Syndrome Association has also done much to provide support and to help in the destigmatisation of people born with the syndrome.

Life expectancy and effects of ageing in people with Down's syndrome

A striking development over the last few decades has been the significant improvement in the life expectancy of people with Down's syndrome from less than ten years in the early 1900s to a mean life expectancy of nearly 50 years today (Malone 1988; Penrose 1949). With changes in social policy this has also generally been accompanied by greater educational and employment opportunities and a more varied and interesting quality of life in adulthood. However, with this increase in life expectancy the potential problems which may occur in older age have become of greater significance. Whereas congenital disorders soon become apparent at birth, these other problems may present insidiously later in life, and knowing about the potential for their development is therefore important in increasing the chance of detection and, if possible, treatment.

Although life expectancy has significantly improved it is still below that of the general population. The reason for this is unknown but it has been argued that people with Down's syndrome age prematurely and the problems which are to be expected in old age occur in Down's syndrome in the fourth and fifth decade of life (Martin 1978). This includes increased rates of visual impairments due to cataract formation, hearing impairments and thyroid disorders. Over 30 per cent of people with Down's syndrome over the age of 40 may have an underactive thyroid gland (Prasher 1995), some presenting with the resultant weight increase, physical and mental slowing, and skin and hair changes characteristic of hypothyroidism. This is an easily treatable condition and these problems correct themselves following daily replacement with thyroxine (Thase 1982). In addition to these observations it has been known since the early 1900s that people with Down's syndrome almost invariably develop changes in their brains with increasing age which are almost identical to those which are now considered to be characteristic of dementia due to Alzheimer's disease (Jervis 1948; Malamud 1964; see Mann 1993 for a review). Studies of the brains of people with Down's syndrome who have died in childhood or in later life have shown that there is increased deposition of the amyloid protein (characteristically found in Alzheimer's disease) in the brain from early in life (Teller *et al.* 1996) and certainly before ten years of age, and by 30 the classical plaques and neurofibrillary tangles of Alzheimer's disease are apparent in the brains of almost all those studied at death (Mann and Esiri 1989). This was not the case for people who had learning disabilities for reasons other than Down's syndrome, suggesting that it was the presence of trisomy 21 which was particularly important and not the non-specific effects of delayed or abnormal brain development resulting from other chromosomal, genetic or environmentally determined reasons. This observation resulted in a search of chromosome 21 for a possible 'candidate gene' which, if inherited in triplicate, might lead to Alzheimer's disease. The gene coding for the amyloid precursor protein (APP) was localised on chromosome 21 (q11–q22) (Goldgaber *et al.* 1987) and, in addition, excess amyloid production in both blood and brain in Down's syndrome was reported (Rumble *et al.* 1989). Subsequently mutations in this gene have been shown to be responsible for certain rare cases of early onset Alzheimer's disease in the general population which is inherited in specific families (Goate *et al.* 1991). Further research on Alzheimer's disease in the general population has reported the presence of mutations in genes located on chromosome 14 in addition to those affecting the APP gene on chromosome 21 (Alzheimer's Disease Collaborative Group 1995). In the case of Down's syndrome these numerous neuropathological studies led, in turn, to more detailed clinical studies asking the question: are these brain changes associated with the impaired memory, the loss of skills and the personality changes characteristic of dementia? (See the reviews in Holland and Oliver 1995; Oliver and Holland 1986).

Cognitive decline and dementia in people with Down's syndrome

While the neuropathological studies suggested that all people with Down's syndrome over 30 years of age had the neuropathological features of Alzheimer's disease, it has been less clear to what extent this resulted in changes in cognitive function with increasing age and ultimately to the classical picture of dementia. Evidence indicating that cognitive decline and eventual dementia does occur is now very compelling, but it is also clear that not everyone with DS is affected (Aylward *et al.* 1995). Early anecdotal case reports described changes with increasing age in people with Down's syndrome which had all the characteristics of dementia. These are summarised in the review by Oliver and Holland (1986). Later studies compared the cognitive and adaptive behaviours of younger versus older people with Down's syndrome, and almost always reported poorer function in the latter group. Such studies were not able to determine whether this was due to cognitive decline with age or to a cohort effect, particularly as the older groups were likely to have had less education in childhood and fewer opportunities in adult life. Comparisons of younger versus older people with Down's syndrome and also comparisons with matched groups without Down's syndrome found age-related impairments in new long-term memory and visuospatial construction specific to Down's syndrome (Haxby 1989; Thase 1984).

Interpretation of these findings has also been difficult because of the marked variation in cognitive abilities across the Down's syndrome population, and a poor score on a specific test of cognitive ability may reflect either the presence of the long-standing learning disability, the presence of dementia or a combination of both. Dementia is characterised by changes in a number of domains of cognitive abilities which in turn affect functioning. Therefore the diagnosis in people with pre-existing learning disabilities can be problematic. The diagnostic features of dementia include the development of impairments in the following: language (aphasias); the ability to perform complex tasks (apraxias); memory; disorientation; the loss of everyday skills; and changes in personality (see World Health Organisation 1992 ICD 10 criteria, and American Psychiatric Association 1994 DSM IV criteria). For dementia to be diagnosed these changes have to be due to an organically determined cause and not due to a transient delirium. As described earlier, visual and hearing impairments are common with increasing age (Evenhuis 1995a, b), and other psychiatric disorders, common in older people and which can mimic dementia, also occur, such as depression (Burt, Loveland and Lewis 1992). The lifestyle of older people with Down's syndrome, particularly in more institutional settings, may be relatively undemanding. The basic skills of living such as cooking and travelling on public transport thus may never have been acquired and therefore loss, due to the onset of dementia, is not apparent.

There have been no truly population-based epidemiological studies using established interview schedules and internationally recognised criteria investigating the prevalence and incidence of dementia in Down's syndrome. Such studies are particularly important to determine service need. Those studies which have been undertaken have reported rates of dementia of 8 per cent in those aged between 35 and 49 years, and between 50 and 75 per cent in those over 60 years (Lai and Williams 1989; Zigman *et al.* 1995). Evenhuis (1990) in a prospective longitudinal study followed 17 older people with Down's syndrome until their death and found that 15 of them developed dementia, with a mean age of onset of 51.3 years in those with previous mild learning disabilities and 52.6 years in those with previously more severe learning disabilities. Such studies as these are now more possible as agreed diagnostic criteria are established for the diagnosis of dementia in people with pre-existing learning disabilities and a range of neuropsychological tests to measure different areas of cognitive function are readily available (Aylward *et al.* 1995; Janicki *et al.* 1995).

The findings of these clinical studies indicating that the Alzheimer-like neuropathological changes almost universal in people with Down's syndrome are associated with the clinical features of dementia, are also supported by studies using different forms of brain imaging. In essence, studies of brain structure, function and neuronal breakdown indicate cerebral atrophy, developing patterns of impaired brain function and neuronal loss, certainly in the fourth and fifth decades of life, in a significant proportion of people with Down's syndrome (Kesslak *et al.* 1994; Murata *et al.* 1993; Schapiro, Haxby and Grady 1992; Schapiro *et al.* 1989).

Risk factors and reasons for cognitive decline and dementia with age in people with Down's syndrome

As yet the identification of those factors which might increase or decrease the risk of cognitive decline and dementia with increasing age in people with Down's syndrome is a relatively unexplored area, yet it is potentially of great importance. Studies in the general population have taken a lead in this area. The most striking risk factor for dementia in both the general population and in Down's syndrome is increasing age. In the case of the former, prevalence rates of dementia increase from under 2 per cent in those aged 65–70 years to 10 per cent in those over 85, with incidence rates of 2.3 per cent in those of 75–80 years and an approximate doubling with every five years' increase in the age group (Paykel *et al.* 1994). A previous history of depression, the presence of a thyroid disorder and a history of past head injury further increase the risk (Van

Duijin and Hofman 1992). Two other factors have been established as being of particular importance in the general population. These are, first, the presence of a family history of dementia of the Alzheimer type in first degree relatives (Heston *et al.* 1981) and, second, the influence of variations in a specific gene called ApoE. The inheritance of particular types of that gene has an effect in the general population and the likelihood of developing Alzheimer's disease. It seems also to have an effect possibly on life expectancy in people with Down's syndrome (Mann 1995).

Systematic studies of the effects of the level of pre-existing learning disability, previous education and lifestyle on the risk and age of onset of dementia in people with Down's syndrome have not been undertaken. One concept of Alzheimer's disease is that the age of onset may depend upon the 'reserve capacity' of the brain. Those with less reserve capacity present sooner with the clinical consequences (that is, cognitive decline and dementia) of the neuropathological process which affects brain function. If this is the case, then people with Down's syndrome who have had a greater degree of learning disability might be expected to have an earlier age of onset and an even higher rate of dementia. This is not supported by the data of Evenhuis (1990), but more systematic studies are required.

Research in this area needs to focus not only on possible environmental and biological factors which may influence the risk in Down's syndrome of developing Alzheimer's disease, but also to explore the possible mechanisms which might explain the relationship between these two disorders. While the increased production of amyloid consequent upon the presence of three copies of the APP gene is likely to be important, the role of 'hydroxyl radicals' may also be of significance. The gene for superoxide dismutase is also on chromosome 21, and the increased activity of this enzyme results in increased production of potentially damaging hydroxyl radicals (Brooksbank and Balaz 1988). Two recent studies, one using cultured trisomy 21 neuronal cells (Busciglio and Yankner 1996) and the other based on animal research (Thomas *et al.* 1996), give some support to this hypothesis. The importance of such theories is that they lead to testable hypotheses and to the potential for the use of preventive treatments. For example, if hydroxyl radical damage was shown to be an important predisposing or causative factor for Alzheimer's disease in Down's syndrome then the use of anti-oxidants such as vitamin E may give some protection. Indirect support for this has been found in one clinical study of aged-matched subjects with Down's syndrome with and without dementia. Those with dementia had significantly lower serum vitamin E levels (Jackson *et al.* 1988). Such observations require further investigation but illustrate how mainstream Alzheimer's disease research may have important implications for the study of ageing in people with Down's syndrome.

Differential diagnosis of decline in older people with Down's syndrome

There are potentially two serious errors which can occur when faced with evidence of apparent cognitive decline in a person with Down's syndrome. The first is that the presence of decline is not recognised when it is occurring. The apparent inability of an older person with Down's syndrome to undertake a particular task is simply written off as 'due to their learning disability'. Sadly there are all too frequently situations where there is a lack of reliable past information about a person because they are unable to give that information themselves and contact has been lost with their family. This is confounded by frequent changes of paid carers. To make a diagnosis of dementia requires a good knowledge of the person over the previous months or years. The second potential error is to assume that apparent decline in a person with Down's syndrome later in life is necessarily due to Alzheimer's disease. This is a serious error as the cause may be eminently treatable or at least partially remedial. The effects of increasing hearing and/or visual impairments may present with impaired ability, hypothyroidism can present with changes in mental functioning, and depression in older people can mimic dementia. These are all treatable disorders. It is therefore important to establish the diagnosis as certainly as possible. The diagnosis of dementia in a person with a pre-existing learning disability requires evidence of a deterioration in a number of areas of cognitive functioning from an established baseline. Table 6.1 summarises these, based on established DSM IV (American Psychiatric Association 1994) and ICD 10 (World Health Organisation 1992) criteria. Information from a formal carer or family member who has known the person for some time is essential. Structured interview schedules, such as the Cambridge Assessment for Mental Disorders in the Elderly (CAMDEX; Roth *et al.* 1986), can be helpful, and a series of neuropsychological instruments to assess specific areas of cognitive function can be used to assess present abilities and loss of specific functions over time. These can include the following: the Rivermead Behavioural Memory Test (Wilson, Cockburn and Baddeley 1985), standard tests of orientation, visuo-spatial skills, language expression and comprehension such as found in test batteries such as the CAMCOG (Huppert *et al.* 1995) and mini-mental state examination (Aylward *et al.* 1995; Folstein, Folstein and McHugh 1975). These may require modification, and where the person has a pre-existing severe

**Table 6.1: Diagnostic criteria for dementia in people
with learning disabilities**

A. Evidence of deterioration in short- and long-term memory. This includes a deterioration in the ability to learn new information and an inability to remember personal information. It needs to be established that the ability previously existed but has been lost by, for example, using standard tests of memory repeated at six-monthly intervals or by reliable information from informants.

B. At least one of the following (in each case evidence of loss of ability is required either through informants or by the repeated use of standardised tests or assessment schedules):

   1. Evidence of a deterioration in the ability to think and reason. A slowing of mental processes or a deterioration in the ability to describe one's thoughts, feelings and experiences.

   2. Evidence of the development of disturbance of higher cortical function such as aphasias (disorder of language due to brain dysfunction), apraxias (inability to carry out motor activities despite intact comprehension and motor function) and agnosias (failure to recognise or identify objects despite intact sensory function).

   3. Evidence of previously acquired complex living skills; for example, the ability to prepare drinks or meals, to play a particular game or to carry out tasks such as shopping.

   4. Evidence of personality change; for example, alteration or accentuation of previous pre-morbid traits.

C. The loss of cognitive abilities are of sufficient severity to interfere with social or occupational functioning.

D. State of consciousness is not clouded (i.e. does not meet the criteria for delirium or intoxication).

At least G and either E or F:

**Table 6.1: Diagnostic criteria for dementia in people
with learning disabilities (continued)**

E. Evidence from the history, physical examination or on investigation of
specific organic factors that is judged to be aetiologically related to the
disturbance. For example, the recent onset of seizures suggestive of
the development of an organic brain disorder, evidence of cerebral
atrophy on computer tomography brain scan.

F. In the absence of such evidence, an organic factor necessary for
development of the syndrome can be presumed if conditions other
than organic mental disorder have been reasonably excluded and if
the observed changes represent cognitive changes in a variety of areas.

G. Such factors as sensory impairments or thyroid disorder can be shown
to be absent or, if present, not to be the sole explanation for the
observed change.

learning disability may be of less value as a means of assessing deterioration in
cognitive functioning as the person may already be at the floor of the test.

Conclusions

There is now conclusive evidence that people with Down's syndrome are at
particular risk for developing the characteristic clinical features of dementia in
later life. Numerous neuropathological studies indicate that this is likely to be
due to the development of Alzheimer-like neuropathological changes which
start with amyloid deposition in early life, leading eventually to the classical
Alzheimer features of plaques and neurofibrillary tangles and ultimately to
cerebral atrophy. Testable hypotheses to account for this association between
a chromosomally determined disorder present from conception on the one
hand, and a disease in later life on the other, are emerging, particularly with
the localisation of the APP gene on chromosome 21. Detailed clini-
cal/neuropathological studies are required to establish the critical cerebral
events which lead to extensive neuronal cell death and thus to the consequences
referred to as 'dementia' (Mukaetova-Ladinska *et al.* 1994).

Clinical studies are not only improving the diagnostic techniques available,
but are establishing reliable estimates of age-dependent prevalence rates of
both cognitive decline and dementia in people with Down's syndrome. Other

factors which can contribute to or mimic dementia are known and the clinical task is to ensure that an accurate diagnosis is established. When dementia is present this is only the beginning of the task of making sure that appropriate care is provided which can adapt to the changing abilities of the person concerned and, in turn, helps to maintain a dignified quality of life and which keeps the carers informed and supported (Holland, Karlinsky and Berg 1993; McCreary *et al.* 1993). Increasingly organisations for people with Down's syndrome are recognising the significance of this association between these two disorders and are themselves publishing information of help to carers (Marler and Cunningham 1995).

Acknowledgement

My thanks to Robbie Patterson for her administrative and secretarial support.

References

Alzheimer's Disease Collaborative Group (1995) 'The structure of the presenilin 1(S182) gene and identification of six novel mutations in early onset AD families.' *Nature Genetics, II*, 219–222.

American Psychiatric Association (1994) *Diagnostic and Statistical Manual of Mental Disorders.* 4th edition. (DSM-IV) Washington DC: American Psychiatric Association.

Aylward, E.H., Burt, D.B., Thorpe, L.U., Lai, F. and Dalton, A.J. (1995) *Diagnosis of Dementia in Individuals with Intellectual Disability.* Washington: American Association on Mental Retardation.

Berg, J.M., Karlinsky, H. and Holland, A.J. (eds) (1993) *Alzheimer Disease, Down Syndrome and their Relationship.* Oxford: Oxford University Press.

Brooksbank, B.W.L. and Balaz, R. (1988) 'Superoxide dismutase and lipoperoxidation in Down's syndrome fetal brain. *Lancet (i),* 88–92.

Burt, D.B., Loveland, K.A. and Lewis, K.R. (1992) 'Depression and the onset of dementia in adults with mental retardation.' *American Journal on Mental Retardation 96,* 502–511.

Busciglio, J. and Yankner, B.A. (1996) 'Apoptosis and increased generation of reactive oxygen species in Down's Syndrome neurons in vitro.' *Nature 378,* 776–779.

Carr, J. (1995) *Down's Syndrome.* Cambridge: Cambridge University Press.

Ciccheti, D. and Beeghley, M. (eds) (1990) *Children with Down Syndrome: A Developmental Perspective.* Cambridge: Cambridge University Press.

Down, J.L. (1866) 'Observations on an ethnic classification of idiots.' *London Hospital, Clinical Lecture and Report 3,* 259–262.

Evenhuis, H.M. (1990) 'The natural history of dementia in Down's Syndrome.' *Archives of Neurology 47*, 263–267.

Evenhuis, H.M. (1995a) 'Medical aspects of ageing in a population with intellectual disability: 1. Visual impairment.' *Journal of Intellectual Disability Research 39*, 1, 19–25.

Evenhuis, H.M. (1995b) 'Medical aspects of ageing in a population with intellectual disability: II. Hearing impairment.' *Journal of Intellectual Disability Research 39*, 1, 27–33.

Flint, J., Wilkie, A.O.M., Buckle, V.J., Winter, R.M., Holland, A.J. and McDermid, H.E. (1995) 'Subtelomeric chromosomal deletions explain a significant fraction of idiopathic mental retardation.' *Nature Genetics 9*, 132–139.

Folstein, M.F., Folstein, S.E. and McHugh, P.R. (1975) 'Mini-Mental State Examination. A practical method for grading the cognitive state of patients for the clinician.' *Journal of Psychiatric Research 12*, 189–198.

Goate, A., Chartier-Harlin, M.-C., Mullan, M., Brown, J., Crawford, F., Fidani, L. *et al.* (1991) 'Segregation of a missense mutation in the amyloid precursor protein gene with familial Alzheimer's disease.' *Nature 349*, 704–706.

Goldgaber, D., Lerman, M.I., MacBride, O.W., Saffioti, U. and Gajdusecek, D.C. (1987) 'Characterisation and chromosomal localisation of a cDNA encoding brain amyloid of Alzheimer's disease.' *Science 235*, 877–880.

Hamerton, J.L. (1982) 'Frequence of mosaicism, translocation, and other variants of trisomy 21.' In F. F. del la Cruz and P.S. Gerald (eds) *Trisomy 21 (Down's Syndrome): Research Perspectives.* Baltimore: University Park Press.

Haxby, J.V. (1989) 'Neuropsychological evaluation of adults with Down's syndrome: patterns of selective impairment in non-demented old adults.' *Journal of Mental Deficiency Research 33*, 193–210.

Heston, L.L., Mastri, A.R., Anderson, A.R. and Anderson, V.E. (1981) 'The genetics of Alzheimer's disease. Association with hematological malignancy and Down's syndrome. *Archives of General Psychiatry 34*, 976–981.

Holland, A.J. and Oliver, C. (1995) 'Down's syndrome and the links with Alzheimer's disease.' *Journal of Neurology, Neurosurgery and Psychiatry 59*, 111–114.

Holland, A.J., Karlinsky, H. and Berg, J.M. (1993) 'Alzheimer disease in persons with Down's syndrome: diagnostic and management considerations.' In J.M. Berg, H. Karlinsky and A.J. Holland (eds) *Alzheimer Disease, Down's Syndrome and their Relationship.* Oxford: Oxford University Press.

Huppert, F.A., Brayne, C., Gill, C., Paykel, E.S. and Beardsall, L. (1995) 'CAMCOG – a concise neuropsychological test to assist dementia diagnosis: socio-demographic determinants in an elderly population sample.' *British Journal of Clinical Psychology 34*, 529–541.

Jackson, C.V.E., Holland, A.J., Williams, C.A. and Dickerson, J.W.T. (1988) 'Vitamin E and Alzheimer's disease in subjects with Down's syndrome.' *Journal of Mental Deficiency Research 32*, 479–484.

Janicki, M.P., Heller, T., Seltzer, G.B. and Hogg, J. (1995) *Practice Guidelines for the Clinical Assessment and Care Management of Alzheimer and other Dementias among Adults with Mental Retardation.* Washington: American Association on Mental Retardation.

Jervis, G.A. (1948) 'Early senile dementia in mongoloid idiocy.' *American Journal of Psychiatry 105,* 102–106.

Kesslak, J.P., Nagata, S.F., Lott, I. and Nalcioglu, O. (1994) 'Magnetic resonance imaging analysis of age-related changes in the brain of individuals with Down's syndrome.' *Neurology 44,* 1039–1045.

Lai, F. and Williams, R.S. (1989) 'A prospective study of Alzheimer's disease in Down's syndrome.' *Archives of Neurology 46,* 849–853.

Lejeune, J., Gautier, M. and Turpin, R. (1959) 'Etudes des chromosomes somatiques de neuf enfants mongliens.' *C.R. Academic Sciences 248,* 1721.

Malamud, N. (1964) 'Neuropathology.' In H.A. Stevens and R. Heber (eds) *Mental Retardation: A Review of Research.* Chicago: University of Chicago Press.

Malone, Q. (1988) 'Mortality and survival of the Down's syndrome population in Western Australia.' *Journal of Mental Deficiency Research 32,* 59–65.

Mann, D.M.A. (1993) 'Association between Alzheimer disease and Down syndrome: neuropathological observations.' In J.M. Berg, H. Karlinsky and A.J. Holland (eds) *Alzheimer Disease, Down Syndrome and their Relationship.* Oxford: Oxford University Press.

Mann, D.M.A. (1995) 'Down's syndrome as a model of the pathological process of Alzheimer's disease.' *Alzheimer's Research 1* (Suppl. 1), 14.

Mann, D.M.A. and Esiri, M.M. (1989) 'The pattern of acquisition of plaques and tangles in Down's syndrome patients under 50 years of age.' *Journal of Neurological Science 89,* 169–179.

Marler, R. and Cunningham, C. (1995) *Down's Syndrome and Alzheimer's Disease.* London: Down's Syndrome Association.

Martin, G. (1978) 'Genetic syndromes in man with potential relevance to pathobiology of ageing.' In D. Bergsman, D.E. Harrison and N.W. Paul (eds) *Genetics Effects of Ageing, Birth Defect, Original Article Series.* New York: The National Foundation – March of Dimes/A.R. Liss, pp. 5–39.

McCreary, B.D., Fotheringham, J.B., Holden, J.J.A., Ouellette-Kuntz, H. and Robertson, D.M. (1993) 'Experiences in an Alzheimer clinic for persons with Down syndrome.' In J.M. Berg, H. Karlinsky and A.J. Holland (eds) *Alzheimer Disease, Down Syndrome and their Relationship.* Oxford: Oxford University Press.

Mukaetova-Ladinska, E., Harrington, C.R., Roth, M. and Wischik, C.M. (1994) 'Distribution of tau protein in Down's syndrome: quantitative differences from Alzheimer's disease.' *Developmental Brain Dysfunction 7,* 311–329.

Murata, T., Koshino, Y. Omorie, *et al.* (1993) 'In vivo proton magnetic resonance spectroscopy study of premature ageing in adults with Down's syndrome.' *Biological Psychiatry 34,* 290–297.

Oliver, C. and Holland, A.J. (1986) 'Down's syndrome and Alzheimer's disease: a review.' *Psychological Medicine 16*, 307–322.

Paykel, E.S., Braynes, C., Huppert, F.A. *et al.* (1994) 'Incidence of dementia in a population older than 75 years in the United Kingdom.' *Archives of General Psychiatry 51*, 325–332.

Penrose, L.S. (1939) 'Maternal age, order of birth and developmental abnormalities.' *Journal of Mental Science 85*, 1141–1150.

Penrose, L.S. (1949) 'The incidence of mongolism in the general population.' *Journal of Mental Science 95*, 685–688.

Prasher, V.P. (1995) 'Age-specific prevalence, thyroid dysfunction and depressive symptomatology in adults with Down's syndrome and dementia.' *International Geriatric Journal of Psychiatry 10*, 25–31.

Roth, M., Huppert, F.A., Tym, E. and Mountjoy, C.Q. (1986) *CAMDEX: The Cambridge Examination for Mental Disorder of the Elderly.* Cambridge: Cambridge University Press.

Rumble, B., Retallack, R., Hilbich, C. *et al.* (1989) 'Amyloid A4 protein and its precursor in Down's syndrome and Alzheimer's disease.' *New England Journal of Medicine 320*, 1446–1452.

Schapiro, M.B., Luxenberg, J.S., Kayes, J.A. *et al.* (1989) 'Serial quantitative CT analysis of brain morphometrics in adults with Down's syndrome with different ages.' *Neurology 39*, 1349–1353.

Schapiro, M.B., Haxby, J.V. and Grady, C.L. (1992) 'Nature of mental retardation and dementia in Down Syndrome: study with PET, CT and neuropsychology.' *Neurobiology of Aging 13*, 723–734.

Teller, J.K., Russo, C., DeBusk, L.M., Angelini, G., Zaccheo, D., Dagna-Bricarelli, F., Scartezzini, P., Bertolini, S., Mann, D.M.A., Tabaton, M. and Gambetti, P. (1996) 'Presence of soluble amyloid ß-peptide precedes amyloid plaques formation in Down's syndrome.' *Nature Medicine 2*, 1, 93–95.

Thase, M.E. (1982) 'Reversible dementia in Down's syndrome.' *Journal of Mental Deficiency Research 26*, 111–113.

Thase, M.E. (1984) 'Age-related neuropsychological deficits in Down's syndrome.' *Biological Psychiatry 4*, 571–585.

Thomas, T., Thomas, G., McLendon, C., Sutton, T. and Mullan, M. (1996) 'ß-amyloid-mediated vasoactivity and vascular endothelial damage.' *Nature 380*, 168–171.

Van Duijin, C.M. and Hofman, A. (1992) 'Risk factors for Alzheimer's disease: the EURODERM collaborative re-analysis of case-control studies.' *Neuroepidemiology 11* (Suppl. 1), 106–113.

Wilson, B., Cockburn, J. and Baddeley, A.D. (1985) *The Rivermead Behavioural Memory Test Reading.* Farham, Hants.: Thames Valley Test Company.

World Health Organisation (1992) ICD-10: *International Statistical Classification of Diseases and Related Health Problems.* 10th revision. Geneva: WHO.

Zigman, W., Schupf, N., Haveman, M. and Silverman, W. (1995) *Epidemiology of Alzheimer Disease in Mental Retardation: Results and Recommendations from an International Conference.* Washington: American Association on Mental Retardation.

PART III
User and Carer Perspectives

Chapter 7

Hearing Their Voice

Malcolm Goldsmith

For many years, mental decline in older people aroused very little interest in the spheres of politics, medicine or social policy. Cognitive failure was seen as being an inevitable part of the ageing process, and the care of elderly people and the study of ageing were not seen as priority areas. They did not attract many people who were advancing their careers, nor did they attract much research funding. The net result of all this was one of neglect (McLean 1987).

After years of relative neglect, dementia is now being seen as an area worthy of study and worthy of funding, and whilst not having the same popular or emotive appeal as AIDS, it is now becoming not only a respectable area of study, but also an attractive one. One of the issues which is now being considered is that of matching services to the needs of people with dementia in ways which the people involved, as well as those who care for them, feel to be appropriate. The idea of asking users what they think about services is not new, and it is being positively pursued in a large number of areas. It is, however, new (and rare!) to ask people suffering from dementia whether they are satisfied with the services they receive, and whether there might be other, more appropriate services which they would like to receive.

Consulting people with dementia

In the Department of Health's *The Health of the Nation* (1992) it is stated quite clearly that people providing services have a duty, 'to consult fully with users and carers in the drawing up and monitoring of community care plans'. The prevailing wisdom in dementia care seems to be that, because of the nature of the illness, it is not possible or practicable to consult with people who have dementia. Indeed it seems to be quite a step forward to involve the family carer in discussions about care, let alone the person with dementia. Wherever studies have been made to test out whether some form of consultation is possible, the conclusion is reached that it is possible. These studies, some of which are referred to below, are few in number, deal with extremely small numbers of people, and the people are probably at a fairly early stage in the development of their illness. Nevertheless, the principle seems to be established that communication about services is possible. The fact that such consultation so rarely seems to happen suggests that once a diagnosis of dementia is made it is then automatically assumed that the person so diagnosed is now incapable of entering into dialogue about their condition and about their hopes and fears.

In 1990 Laura Sutton and Felicity Fincham (1994) investigated how people with mild to moderate communication difficulties viewed and experienced respite care. What became clear was that social factors rather than the physical aspects of care were of greatest importance to them, and the authors concluded that their study, 'cautions against the all too ready assumption that dementia sufferers are too confused or out of touch with reality to offer a users' perspective'.

A study by Lunne Phair published in 1990 described interviews with people using services at one particular centre, and it showed that clients, 'both mentally alert and mentally frail were able to give their perceptions of the unit'. She went on to stress the importance of gaining the viewpoint of mentally confused people because their perception might be different to that of the carers and those giving the service. She argued that it was important for democracy that efforts were made to obtain the views of users of services, and she stressed the importance of ensuring that the views of mentally frail people were elicited. Granted this conviction and determination, she found in her own study that it was in fact possible to obtain their views. As a result, she was able to demonstrate that the clients and carers were pleased with the specific service that they were receiving, and a number of recommendations were made in the light of their comments to ensure the maintenance of the high standard of care and attention that already existed: 'No criticisms from the clients were damning and all suggestions are made to maintain and improve what is proving to be a very good multidisciplinary multifunctional service'.

David Sperlinger and Louise McAuslane (1994) undertook a pilot study of the views of users of services for people with learning difficulties and dementia in a London borough. They interviewed in depth six people in the early stages of dementia, and found that for four of the six people it was clear that there were issues and concerns that they wished to share with the researchers. Although many aspects of care were discussed in the interviews, it was the *social aspects* that were of greater concern to the users than matters relating to food, travel and the environment. The authors conclude that, 'our experience suggests that generally people using these services have plenty to say...it is clear from this pilot study that it is possible to consult with some users of the dementia services in a meaningful way'.

Another study (Lam and Beech 1994) carried out a consultation with both users and carers of a weekend break project, and this again showed that it was possible to engage with people who have dementia and discuss their views of the service. The study concluded that, 'despite a progressive decline in memory and cognitive powers, people with dementia retain the capacity to experience the whole range of emotions, and the capacity to contribute to, and benefit from social relationships'.

A study by Brenda Gillies (1995) focusing on the subjective experience of dementia demonstrated that, although not an easy task, it is possible to interview people with dementia and gain an insight into their views and preferences. She comments that:

> ...this study is one of the first opportunities afforded to dementia sufferers to reflect on their situation and express opinion about how they are supported by those who look after them, both formally and informally. As such, the resulting accounts...should be given due consideration and should be regarded as a unique source of insightful information for those charged with providing quality services to them.

This approach was reinforced by Keady, Nolan and Gilliard (1995) in their study 'Listen to the voices of experience'.

If anyone doubts the possibility of conversing with people with dementia, even in relatively advanced stages, then the account of Valerie Sinason's year-long psychotherapeutic relationship with Edward Johnson (1992) makes compulsive reading, and the detailed sociolinguistic study of Heidi Ehernberger Hamilton (1994) reminds us of just what can be achieved if we combine skill, determination and patience.

Some questions to be asked

It is certainly desirable that we should be able to hear the voice of people with dementia and, if possible, to hear their views about the services which are provided and the services which they would like. The fact that this may be a difficult process, and that it may be impossible with some people, should not mean that we assume that it is impossible with all of them. In my own study (Goldsmith 1996) I interviewed a number of people with dementia and reflected upon the problems that I encountered in that process. To what extent are problems in communication inevitable and a consequence of a person's illness and to what extent are they dependent upon variables which can be addressed, and what is the relationship between the two?

To the question, 'is it desirable to hear their voice?' the answer must be an unqualified 'yes'. To the question, 'is it possible?', the answer must be a qualified 'yes'. We are not yet in a position where we can generally speak easily with people with dementia all of the time, but we know that some people are able to communicate with some people some of the time. The first challenge is to discover ways in which more people might be enabled to communicate more easily with more people for more of the time. The second challenge is, once we have established communication, to act upon what is being communicated. I believe that the first and perhaps the most important step that has to be taken is one of attitude. It is important to develop an approach which seeks to maximise what is still possible, to believe that it may be possible to do more, and to work on the assumption that communication *is* possible to a much later stage than has hitherto been thought. It is then important to devise or develop services to meet the expressed needs of people with dementia. This may mean occasionally adjusting services from meeting what others perceive to be their needs. It requires a certain flexibility of mind and, dare one say it, a certain humility, to be willing to address such issues.

Different approaches

There is a certain degree of tension between what might be called the *biomedical approach* and what might be called the *personhood approach*. The first tends to concentrate upon the physical, and is individualistic and discrete, whilst the second tends to concentrate upon the social, and is more corporate. One might be said to be disease-centred whilst the other is person-centred. Of course, such a simplification does little justice to either position and in actual fact they are complementary and need each other rather than being mutually exclusive. Nevertheless it is a helpful distinction to make in order to help us 'get into' the debate about the nature of dementia. Fontana and Smith (1989) write about the concept of 'unbecoming' and suggest that even when the person with dementia appears to be understanding and communicating there is often less substance and self-awareness than carers are able to admit:

> ...the self has slowly unravelled and 'unbecome' a self, but caregivers take the role of the other and assume that there is a person behind the largely unwitting presentation of self of the victims, albeit in reality there is less

and less, until where once there was a unique individual there is but emptiness (p.45).

The concept of personhood contrasts with this and seeks to see the person within the context of their whole life, their history, their general health, their family structure and social relationships, as well as within the context of their specific neurological impairment. All these things combine to make a person who they are, and to concentrate on one without the others is to treat the person as less than a whole person. This point was illustrated by Michael Ignatieff (1994) when he said:

> I learned as much from my mother when she couldn't speak to me, when she couldn't communicate, when she simply stared and received our kisses on her cheek, as I learned when she was joking and laughing. What she taught me was that it's just an illness. It's a terrible illness, but it's just an illness.

I am labouring this point somewhat, but I think that it is of crucial importance, as Karen Lyman (1989) pointed out, 'in reality, the psycho-social experience of a dementing illness cannot be contained within biomedical concepts of brain disease'.

Marginalisation

Very often the person with dementia is marginalised, and made an 'object' either for studying or for being cared for. There is a tendency for people to withdraw from social relationships with people with dementia, thus making the person even more isolated. The process of disempowering comes both from the course of the disease and from the reactions of other people, so consequently the person with dementia is doubly handicapped. In a much quoted passage Cotrell and Shulz (1993) write:

> In the majority of research on Alzheimer's Disease, the afflicted person is viewed as a disease entity to be studied rather than as someone who can contribute directly to our understanding of the illness and its course...the person with dementia is often relegated to the status of object rather than legitimate contributor to the research process...investigation has focused on cognitive functioning and patient management, with a notable absence of interest in patient awareness and in adaptation to increasing impairment and changing social status as a cause of psychiatric symptoms...one of the most common conditions in Alzheimer's Disease is depression (p.205).

The role of 'the other'

In my own study (Goldsmith 1996) I had to ask myself to what extent did my own limitations and ignorance influence the possibilities of, or obstacles to, communication? This raises the interesting question of what is the role of 'the other' in situations in which people with dementia meet and relate to other people? Kitwood and Bredin (1992) have suggested that perhaps the very idea of 'objectivity' in such relationships, especially where professionals are concerned, is an understandable attempt to distance ourselves from the distress and experience of the reality of dementia:

> Professionals and informal carers are vulnerable people too, bearing their own anxiety and dread concerning frailty, dependence, madness, ageing, dying and death. A supposed objectivity in a context that is, in fact, interpersonal, is one way of maintaining psychological defences, and so making involvement with conditions such as dementia bearable (p.270).

The question that bothered me for so long was why, if we know that communication with people with dementia *is* possible – if not for all, all of the time, certainly for many for much of the time – then why are they so little involved in formulating the patterns of their care? Why are their views apparently so rarely recorded, discussed and taken into consideration? I know that there are a thousand different examples of individual people being listened to, and their care being adjusted to meet their needs, but it all seems to depend, far too often, upon the individual chemistry of the carer and the person with dementia. There seems to be little attempt to gain their views and preferences in any structured sort of way and, certainly in my experience, it seems to be the exception rather than the norm. If this is so, then we need to know why, and we need to find ways of reversing the situation.

Problems to be faced

One of the problems that we have to face when endeavouring to facilitate communication, in the hope of being able to hear people's views about their condition and the services that they receive, is the fact that there are so many variables to be taken into consideration. It is a truism to say that no two people are the same, but when they have dementia it means that a skilled, individual approach is essential. Dementia itself is an umbrella term, used to describe one or more of a whole number of different illnesses, and we need to know much more about the social consequences and implications of each specific illness. It is far from clear whether different dementing illnesses require particular sorts of care and social provision, and whether the process of communication needs to be addressed in different ways. We know how Alzheimer's disease affects speech patterns (Griffiths 1991; Lee 1991), but we know much less about how other forms of dementia affect them. Most of the care packages lump people together under the name 'dementia', with little reference as to how different diseases may have different patterns or to the age or background of the people concerned. Much more work needs to be done in enabling us to understand better the pattern and process of differing types of illness, and of how these affect people's ability to reflect and communicate.

We have people with different personalities, being afflicted by different illnesses (though described by the general name), and needing a whole variety of different services. We also need to know more about, and understand better, the relationships that they have with their family and the whole network of relationships that they bring with them into the experience of dementia. Few assumptions can be made about what kind of support particular individuals and their families need, and therefore there is a great need for us to find ways of knowing what their views are.

What 'works' with one person will not necessarily 'work' with another, and we need to find ways of being able to discern more easily what might be an appropriate service or approach. Knowing a person's life story is an invaluable aid in this process. Mills and Chapman (1992) observed that:

> ...many of us who work with confused elderly people would agree that our knowledge of their past lives, as opposed to the diagnosis and progress of their illness, is inclined to be somewhat sparse...if these patients are seen as the sum total of their problems then the outlook is bleak. We need to see the person behind the dementia (p.27).

A consultant psychiatrist wrote to me saying that he was, 'appalled by the lack of *personal* knowledge about some old people with dementia in residential and nursing homes', and yet we know that knowledge of a person's past is an invaluable help in communicating with them in the present. An American study (Pietrukowicz and Johnson 1991) has shown how staff in a nursing home who had read the life history of residents thought that the residents were more capable of interacting with others, contributing socially and setting goals and adapting than did the staff who had not read their life histories. Knowledge of the narrative is knowledge of the other, knowledge of a person goes a long way towards understanding, and understanding is an enormous help in the process of communication. Build upon flimsy foundations and the edifice can easily and quickly crumble. Charles Murphy (1994) has written a helpful introduction to the use of life histories, and stresses that what is important is what the person wishes to share with us, even if we cannot at the moment fully understand the images or the information which are offered. Faith Gibson (1991, 1994) has written widely about the importance of reminiscence: '...it is wide-ranging and critical. It emphasises the importance of communication, if being able to tell one's own unique life story and have it heeded and respected by others'.

A clinical neuropsychologist wrote saying that the most exciting outcome of knowing a person's life story may be the use of previous experiences and reminiscence about them to establish views on current decisions. Moreover, finding out about family traditions and rituals from the past could allow the re-creation of those traditions in the present. This is an echo of Cotrell and Lein (1993) who observed that:

> ...behaviour may have antecedents in the victim's less impaired history...by introducing a psychological perspective into what has been predomi- nantly a biomedical experience, we may be able to identify factors that hinder or enhance the successful adaptation of the individual to the dementing illness...indeed, we may find that much of the variability in the progression of the disease can be accounted for by psychosocial differences (p.128).

They interpret behavioural disturbances as adaptive attempts to avoid confron- tation with the reality of existing intellectual deficits, and suggest that this often takes place in collusion with the care-giver. Knowing the background of a person, knowing their family context, can be a considerable help in under- standing their present situation, and understanding that can be a great help in the process of communication and hearing their views.

A residential home that I visited on a regular basis had deep chairs around the walls of a large room. No matter what time of day I was there the radio was always on, and sometimes it competed with a television. I was seldom aware of anyone ever watching the television or listening to the radio, they were just on, and they were as much a part of the place as were the chairs and the cigarette smoke. It was whilst reflecting on my visits there that I came to realise the importance that the environment has on our ability to communicate with people with dementia. Visiting people at different times of the day has also alerted me to the fact that the same person may be understandable one day at one time, and yet apparently completely unreachable at a different time on a different day or even on the same day. If we are to hear the voice of people with dementia then we need to pay particular attention to the environment in which we seek to communicate.

In one of the most telling observations sent to me a project manager wrote:

> ...this might seem a daft thing to say but is it not common sense to assume that by removing someone from their own home and placing them in a strange ward, full of strange people and routines, to assess their level of confusion, you will discover a very confused person?

Where we meet people, in what context and in whose company, why we are meeting them, and how we are meeting them are all factors which may affect a person's ability to communicate. The lighting, the colours, the sound level, the warmth (both literal and metaphorical), and the time that we spend with them – all combine to enhance or frustrate the possibilities of them being able to express their voice and of us being able to hear it, and interpret and understand it.

Non-verbal communication

There are many different ways in which people communicate, and speech is not an essential requirement of them all. We are aware of the fact that blind people often seem to have heightened awareness of sound, and they seem to have compensated in some way for their loss of one faculty by developing others to a finer degree. It may well be that, for people with dementia, there are non-verbal ways of communicating that have been heightened and developed. It is all the more frustrating, therefore, if other people are not able to pick up these signals because they are not aware of them and do not expect them. There seems to be a growing amount of evidence to suggest that touch is of great importance, and that we need to find ways of developing opportunities for mutual touching and for interpreting and understanding the significance of touch. Massage, holding hands, hugs, kisses and strokes can all be vehicles for communication. As one person wrote to me: 'I can communicate a great deal by the way that I hold a person's hand. And I believe I can tell a great deal about their emotional state by the pressure exerted in return. Eye contact, tone of voice and body posture are also key components of communication'. We need to find ways of 'hearing the voice' through non-verbal expression, and to recognise this as being valid and meaningful.

Art, music and drama are also ways of empowering people, and enabling them to express their fears and hopes. A paper given at the Alzheimer's Disease International Conference in Edinburgh in 1994 described the work of a drama therapist (Crimmens 1994):

...one of the things we worked really hard to create and reinforce with virtually everything we did was the opportunity for people to be individuals with their needs and preferences respected...offering choice and initiative is a major theme in Drama therapy...a common misconception is that the elderly person who is dementing cannot make choices. I work on the belief that they can and it is up to me to take the time to interpret that person's wishes as accurately and as sensitively as I can.

Time and pace

It is up to me to take the time – and this is the crux of the matter. Communicating with people with dementia requires respect for their sense of time and pace, and it cannot be rushed. This can be quite problematic for those who have to provide services, for they are often driven by busy diaries, targets and external demands placed upon them, and these can be in conflict with the need to move slowly, to have time and, above all, patience. One person commented to me: '...rushing any conversation with a person with dementia, or rushing off when you know they haven't understood without coming back to clarify the statement is tantamount to abuse'. This is another way of expressing Tom Kitwood's (1990) view that, 'we need to slow down our thought processes, to become inwardly quiet, and to have a kind of poetic awareness; that is, to look for the significance of metaphor and allusion rather than pursuing meaning with a kind of relentless tunnel vision' (p.51).

Many staff involved in service provision feel themselves to be under a great deal of pressure, and this can often lead to a situation in which demoralisation and failure are experienced. There is a need for a greater commitment to training in the area of communication. Knowing that they are embarking upon a difficult but important process, which requires skills which can be learned, can help to make work both challenging and satisfying. However, this will only happen if there is a development plan which places an emphasis upon the importance of communication and if management ensures that resources, especially time, are committed to the process. We need to discover the art of creative listening, and we need to move at the time and pace of the person with dementia and not impose our agenda onto them.

Challenging behaviour

Once communication is seen as being important, then we are more likely to be looking for examples of good communication and for hints or suggestions of communication even from people in advanced stages of their illness. A consultant psychiatrist wrote to me saying that when people are not heard then they may become irritable or aggressive, and he quoted Martin Luther King, who said that, 'violence is the voice of the unheard'. There is a growing body of opinion which now regards the challenging behaviour of many people with dementia as being an attempt to communicate something of their frustration and despair. This is an area of study which has been sadly neglected, a point brought out by Teri and others (Teri *et al.* 1992).

The deputy manager of a home for elderly people feels that there is a real challenge to staff to care for people whose behaviour can be very disruptive, and wrote to me saying: 'I am increasingly feeling that any behaviour that we either don't understand or find difficult must be interpreted. I spend a lot of time with staff saying "what else might this mean?"'. It has been suggested that people with dementia try to behave logically, but the challenge is to tap into that logic. This was a point made to me by a clinical psychologist who wrote:

> ...my experience with other client groups tells me that 'bad' behaviour is likely to be an expression of fear, anger or frustration, or is a valid response to the way that the world is perceived by the individual. The notion of the behaviour being a valid response to the phenomenal world of the individual seems particularly interesting as it seems likely that he is 'misperceiving' (by our criteria) his environment. Do we know much yet about the generalities (if any) or individual concepts/perceptions of their immediate world?

Aggressive or violent behaviour, persistent wandering, inappropriate sexual advances and other forms of challenging behaviour can pose real problems for carers and for staff providing services. It is important to find ways of understanding what lies behind such behaviour, and ways of interpreting what it might mean. There is an understandable desire on the part of many people merely to manage and control the behaviour, often by drugs, and whilst this may calm the person down and relieve the stress and anxiety of those around, it does not address the root issue of what is the cause, why does the person behave in this way rather than that way; nor does it seek to understand the behaviour as perhaps an attempt at communication. There is a need for much more work to be done in this area.

Conclusion

Two common misperceptions are made when talking about hearing the voice of people with dementia: the first is that you cannot hear that voice because the very nature of their illness means that they are unable to reflect or to communicate; and the second is that we know what they mean to communicate because without realising it we coax or cajole them to react to us in certain ways so that they give us the information that they think we want to hear. Hearing the views of people with dementia can be a very difficult and taxing job, and those who have that responsibility need a great deal of time, patience and skill. In terms of service provision the implications are extremely far-reaching. If we really believe that it is possible to communicate with people, even during the advanced stages of their illness, and if we also believe that it is desirable that we do so, then there would need to be a considerable shift in the deployment of resources. That is a decision which we need to face up to, and take. It is no answer to avoid it by suggesting that it is not possible to hear the voice of people with dementia, because it clearly is possible, and on a scale which is far beyond that which prevails today in most areas of service provision.

References

Cotrell, V. and Lein, L. (1993) 'Awareness and denial in the Alzheimer's disease victim.' *Journal of Gerontological Social Work 19*, 3/4, 128.

Cotrell, V. and Schulz, R. (1993) 'The perspective of the patient with Alzheimer's disease; a neglected dimension of dementia research.' *The Gerontologist 33*, 205.

Crimmens, P. (1994) 'Drama therapy in the care of people with dementia.' Paper given at the 1994 Alzheimer's Disease International Conference, Edinburgh.

Department of Health (1992) *The Health of the Nation*. London: HMSO.

Fontana, A. and Smith, R. (1989) 'Alzheimer's disease victims: the "unbecoming" of self and the normalization of competence.' *Sociological Perspectives 32*, 1, 45.

Gibson, F. (1991) 'The lost ones: recovering the past to help their present.' Paper given at a BASW study day in Belfast and subsequently published by the Dementia Services Development Centre, University of Stirling.

Gibson, F. (1994) *Reminiscence and Recall*. London: Age Concern.

Gillies, B. (1995) 'The subjective experience of dementia: a qualitative analysis of interviews with dementia sufferers and their carers, and the implications for service provision.' Obtainable from the Department of Medicine, the University of Dundee.

Goldsmith, M. (1996) *Hearing the Voice of People with Dementia: Opportunities and Obstacles*. London: Jessica Kingsley Publishers.

Griffiths, H. (1991) 'The psychiatry of old age: the effects of dementia on communication.' In Gravell and Francis (eds) *Speech and Communication Problems in Psychiatry*. London: Chapman and Hall.

Hamilton, H.E. (1994) *Conversations with an Alzheimer's Patient*. Cambridge: Cambridge University Press.

Ignatieff, M. (1994) quoted in a BBC Radio 4 discussion *All in the Mind*.

Keady, J., Nolan, M. and Gilliard, J. (1995) 'Listen to the voices of experience.' *Journal of Dementia Care* May/June, 15.

Kitwood, T. (1990) 'Psychotherapy and dementia.' *BPS Psychotherapy Section Newsletter 8*.

Kitwood, T. and Bredin, K. (1992) 'Towards a theory of dementia care: personhood and well-being.' *Ageing and Society. 12*, 3, 269–288.

Lam, J. and Beech, L. (1994) 'I'm sorry to go home: the Weekend Break Project: consultation with users and their carers.' Obtainable from Department of Psychology, St. Helier NHS Trust, Sutton Hospital, Cotswold Road, Sutton, Surrey SM2 5NF.

Lee, V. (1991) 'Language changes in Alzheimer's disease: a literature review.' *Journal of Gerontological Nursing 17*, 1.

Lyman, K. (1989) 'Bringing the social back in: a critique of the biomedicalization of dementia.' *The Gerontologist 1*, 29, 5, 600.

McLean, S. (1987) 'Assessing dementia: Part 1: difficulties, definitions and differential diagnosis.' *Australian and New Zealand Journal of Psychiatry 21*, 142–174.

Mills, M. and Chapman, I. (1992) 'Understanding the story.' *Nursing the Elderly 14*, 5, Nov./Dec., 27.

Murphy, C. (1994) *It Started with a Sea-Shell: Life Story Work and People with Dementia*. Stirling: Dementia Services Development Centre, University of Stirling.

Phair, L. (1990) 'What the people think: Homefield Place from the client's point of view.' Obtainable from Eastbourne and County Healthcare, Seaford Day Hospital, Sutton Road, Seaford, East Sussex.

Pietrukowicz, M. and Johnson, M. (1991) 'Using life histories to individualise nursing home staff attitudes towards residents.' *The Gerontologist 31*, 1.

Sinason, V. (1992) 'The man who was losing his brain.' In *Mental Handicap and the Human Condition*. London: Free Association Books.

Sperlinger, D. and McAuslane, L. (1994) 'I don't want you to think I'm ungrateful...but it doesn't satisfy what I want.' Obtainable from Department of

Psychology, St. Helier NHS Trust, Sutton Hospital, Cotswold Road, Sutton, Surrey SM2 5NF.

Sutton, L. and Fincham, F. (1994) 'Clients' perspectives: experiences of respite care.' *PSIG Newsletter 49*.

Teri, L., Rabins, P., Whitehouse, P., Berg, L., Reisberg, B., Sunderland, T., Eichelman, B. and Phelps, C. (1992) 'Management of behaviour disturbance in Alzheimer's disease: current knowledge and future direction.' *Alzheimer Disease and Associated Disorders 6*, 2, 86.

Chapter 8

Coping with Caring for a Person with Dementia

Gillian Parker

Introduction

The past 20 years have seen a burgeoning of interest in the topic of 'informal carers' – those family members, friends and neighbours who support disabled and older people and enable them to live at home. This interest, both in research and in policy, led to support for carers being included as a specific objective of the community care reforms ushered in by the 1990 NHS and Community Care Act.

Research has shown the substantial levels of support that the most heavily involved carers provide and the impact that this has on their lives (Parker and Lawton 1994). Employment, household and personal finances, emotional health, social and family life have all been shown to be affected (Parker 1990). However, of all the caring situations in which people may find themselves, caring for a person with dementia is probably experienced as the most difficult. The symptoms of the condition itself make caring difficult. Dealing with incontinence, wandering, aggressive or dangerous behaviour, sleep disturbance and the need for constant supervision may be added to the support required because of physical impairment. In particular, 'demand' on the attention or emotions of the carer, combined with the 'loss' of the person previously known to the carer because of changed behaviour and personality (Williams, Briggs and Coleman 1995) can make caring both burdensome and unrewarding.

At the same time, the characteristics of people caring for those with dementia may make them less well able to cope with these demands. Because of the late onset of dementia, carers are older on average than other carers and, consequently, in poorer health. A study of dementia sufferers in Liverpool, for example, found that the average age of women caring for husbands was 76 and of men caring for wives, 86. Even carers of a younger generation were nearing retirement age; the average ages of daughters and sons who were carers were 59 and 56, respectively (Wenger 1994). Carers of dementia sufferers are also more likely to be married to the person they care for and, therefore, to live in the same household (Levin, Sinclair and Gorbach 1989; Wenger 1994). This, too, can increase the demands of care-giving.

Most dementia sufferers live at home with the support of informal carers, whether married or not. There is general agreement in the research literature about the behaviours that carers of dementia sufferers find problematic; incontinence, over-demanding behaviour and the need for constant supervision are themes that run through many research papers (see Morris, Morris and Briton 1988 for a review). Further, there is general agreement that the carers of dementia sufferers experience higher levels of 'stress' than people in the general population. However, the relationship between the characteristics of carers and the people they care for, the 'problems' that sufferers present to carers, any stress or psychological problems that the carers may experience and the effect that this may have on eventual outcomes is not immediately clear. This chapter attempts to unravel some of these relationships and the suggestions for supporting carers that follow from them.

The research literature on this topic is now very large. To restrict the ground covered, and to increase its relevance for UK readers, this chapter reviews research from the UK and from Canada and Australia (which have broadly similar approaches to health and social care as the UK). Important early studies from the UK and other research carried out since 1990 are included.

Accounting for carers' stress

Gilhooly (1984) in an early study which examined carers' stress, was unable to identify any aspect of the dementia sufferer's behaviour or personality which influenced the carer's stress levels. By contrast, other research has identified several factors. Isaacs, Livingstone and Neville (1972), for example, suggested that the underlying personality of the sufferer, distortions of personality and behaviour caused by the dementia, and, to a lesser extent, the physical burden of caring made caring 'overwhelming'. More statistically sophisticated work looked at the inter-relationships between the mood states of carers and problems experienced while caring (Gilleard, Watt and Boyd 1981). Five dimensions or factors were identified: dependency, disturbance, disability, demand and wandering. The 'demand' factor – such as repetitive questioning, attention-seeking, disrupting the carer's social life and creating personality clashes – contributed most to carers' reported levels of strain. Once this had been allowed for, none of the other factors contributed significantly to perceived stress. Levin, Sinclair and Gorbach (1983) found a relationship between severe incontinence, trying behaviour, night disturbance and the sufferer's inability to converse normally and carers' high stress scores. Restrictions on the carer's own leisure activities and the time that could be spent with friends and families – problems associated with Gilleard *et al.'s* 'demand' factor – were also important.

As Morris *et al.* (1988) have concluded, there is, 'a broad agreement between studies concerning what behavioural alterations are more likely to be reported as problems: ...the main factors seem to be incontinence, over-demanding behaviour and the need for constant supervision' (p.149). However, there is less agreement on the relationship between these and carers' 'strain' or distress. Some discrepancies, they suggest, 'may reflect the complex relationship between problem behaviour and strain or emotional disturbance in the caregiver...It may be necessary to take into account other aspects, such as the social context of caregiving and the relationship between the caregiver and the sufferer' (p.150).

Attempts to isolate such 'social' factors have been little more successful, with contradictory or inconclusive findings. For example, one of the earliest British studies of dementia (Isaacs *et al.* 1972) suggested that both the age and level of dependency of the sufferer and the age of the carer influenced the carers' experience of stress. More recent work (Ballard *et al.* 1995) similarly found increasing carer age and severity of cognitive impairment significantly associated with depression in carers living with a sufferer (but not in those living elsewhere). By contrast, other work has failed to find any relationship between age of either sufferers or their carers and stress (Levin *et al.* 1983), while Gilleard *et al.* (1984) suggested that older carers experience *less* strain than younger ones.

Similarly, sex of the main carer and sufferer and the relationship between them are related to carers' stress in some studies but not in others. Gilhooly (1983, 1984), for example, found that the *only* sufferers' characteristic significantly associated with the carers' morale was their sex. Those caring for women had better morale and better mental health than those caring for men, a finding replicated by Gilleard *et al.* (1984). The carer's sex can also be important; male carers of dementia sufferers have been shown in several studies to have higher morale (Gilhooly 1984; Levin *et al.* 1983; Morris *et al.* 1991). Some studies suggest that closeness of the kin relationship between the carer and the person they look after influences stress – the more distant the relationship the better the carer's mental health (Gilhooly 1984). Other studies have failed to identify this relationship (Levin *et al.* 1983).

The methods and analysis used may be part of the problem here. Projects do not always control for the inter-relationships of variables that may in themselves, or in combination, affect stress levels. For example, age and sex of the carer, the kin relationship between carer and sufferer, the age and sex of the sufferer and his or her level of dependency are all potentially inter-related. Their impact on stress, whether singly or in combination, cannot be measured without controlling for the effects of the others.

A second problem with the research literature is what is actually being measured. Studies refer variously to stress, burden, lowered morale, depression and psychiatric morbidity; are all these things aspects of the same underlying factor or are they separate factors with different relationships to the caring experience? Even when the terms are the same (for example, 'stress'), different tests are often used to measure them.

Third, there is frequent confusion about the direction of the relationship between 'stress' and the carer and sufferer characteristics. For example, the sufferer's disturbed behaviour may *cause* stress, it may be influenced by the carer's stress, it may make stress easier or harder to deal with, a stressed carer may be more likely to report disturbed behaviour or, indeed, all four may be happening simultaneously.

Because of this confusion, and the failure to identify unequivocal, causal relationships between carer stress and the social and clinical characteristics of their situation (both in relation to dementia and other impairments), some researchers have begun to question the usefulness of further aetiological research of this sort. Carers, as a group, undoubtedly experience higher levels of stress, as measured by the instruments available, than the rest of the population. However, many intuitively plausible factors that might cause higher levels of stress in some carers have not been firmly identified. A more productive approach, it has been suggested, is to emphasise the fact that carers do cope with and adapt to the stress they experience and to attempt to discover how they do it (Byrne and Cunningham 1985). In other words, we might be better employed trying to identify what factors *mediate* the experience of stress and enable carers to cope more or less successfully. Such an approach is in line with recent debate about the ways in which individuals manage threats to their personal welfare (Titterton 1992).

What helps carers to cope?

There are four broad sets of factors which may ameliorate the impact of stress and/or help carers to cope: how carers 'interpret' or 'appraise' caring and the sufferer's condition; the quality of relationship with the sufferer; strategies for dealing with the demands of caring; and relationships with other sources of formal and informal support.

Interpretation and appraisal

One of the most interesting themes to emerge from recent literature in this field is the importance of carers' interpretation of their circumstances (Morris *et al.* 1988). For example, Levesque, Cossette and Laurin (1995) asked carers both about the level or severity of the sufferers' impairment and behaviour problems and about the degree to which they found it 'disturbing'. For certain impairments and behaviours (problems with activities of daily living, depressive behaviour and memory problems) it was carers' feeling more or less disturbed by, rather than the level or severity of, these problems that was related to poorer psychological well-being. By contrast, however, the frequency of *disruptive* behaviour was more closely linked to psychological well-being than was the extent to which it disturbed carers. The authors comment that:

> The difference may be explained by the fact that disruptive behaviors...are potentially dangerous for the relative, the caregiver and sometimes for both; their frequency may therefore be the important aspect. In contrast, functional impairment, memory-related behaviors, and depressive behaviors may provoke sadness as well as annoyance...such reactions may reflect the caregivers' response to the changing relationship with their demented relative. (p.350)

Similarly, Hadjistavropoulos *et al.* (1994) found that while objective measures of sufferers' functioning did not predict care-giver burden, 'the caregivers' *perceptions* [my emphasis] of the patients' everyday functioning and dysphoria influenced burden directly' (p.312). They conclude that, '[o]bjective patient deficits are not directly predictive of caregiver burden whereas the caregivers' assessments of the severity of these deficits are' (p.313). This is a finding echoed in much other work in the area (Morris *et al.* 1988).

Carers' understanding or beliefs about the cause of behavioural problems in the sufferer also seem to influence stress. Those who attribute the problems to, 'laziness or voluntary uncooperativeness and interpret these behaviours as personal assaults or ungratefulness for the care provided' may experience caring as more stressful than carers who attribute other meanings to the behaviour (Levesque *et al.* 1995, p.336).

How carers perceive or interpret caring may be related to their sex. Female carers of dementia sufferers have been shown consistently to experience higher levels of stress than male carers, even when any higher objective burden has been taken into account (Morris *et al.* 1991). It is suggested that this is because men and women both perceive and experience caring differently.

The quality of the relationship between carer and sufferer
Another theme running through the literature is the importance of the quality of the relationship between the carer and the sufferer. Generally, distance in the kin relationship influences the impact on carers' mental health, but this can be cut across by the quality of the relationship. So, 'paradoxically, *within* the relationship, the closer the emotional bond, the *less* is the strain for the caregiver' (Morris *et al.* 1988, pp.150–151, original emphasis). For those caring for spouses, the quality of their marital relationship before the onset of dementia appears to affect whether or not they become depressed (Ballard *et al.* 1995; Morris *et al.* 1988). There is also some suggestion that a high level of conflict in the relationship may be related to acute deterioration in the sufferer and subsequent requests for services. Kitwood (cited by Orrell and Bebbington, 1995, p.314) argues that, 'when self-esteem is damaged by "malignant social psychology" the individual falls into a cycle of discouragement and failure and this occurs when others treat the sufferer in a detrimental way'. Orrell and Bebbington then go on to suggest that their and other studies:

> ...indicate that negative communication in the relationship between the dementia sufferer and carer makes the caring process more difficult. This is because it can lower carers' morale, increase the feeling of stress and burden and possibly lead to poorer patient outcome in terms of worsening problems or an increased likelihood of psychiatric admission. (p.321)

The quality of the relationship has also been explored through examining the level of 'expressed emotion' (EE) displayed by carers. This refers to the frequency of critical comments made by family members about the sufferer and the levels of hostility or emotional involvement they show (Scazufca and Kuipers 1996). The concept has been used extensively and successfully in studies of adults with mental health problems, particularly schizophrenia (Vaughan and Leff 1976) but less so in relation to dementia. Gilhooly and Whittick (1989) measured EE in carers of dementia sufferers and found that it was related both to the quality of the relationship between the sufferer and the carer and to the carer's own well-being, as well as to the carer's contact with friends. As in studies of adult mental health, EE was related to the carers' sex (women have higher levels) but not to the sufferers' level of impairment, sex or age. This suggests a constellation of factors around the quality and dynamics of the relationship that make the experience of caring more or less bearable. However, as Gilhooly and Whittick caution, '[w]e have no way of knowing if high EE causes low morale, and has a negative impact on supporters' mental health, or if low morale and poor mental health cause supporters to be more hostile towards their dementing dependants' (p.270).

Feeling that the person being cared for appreciates the carer's efforts is another aspect of the relationship identified as important in helping carers to cope (Levesque *et al.*1995; Wenger 1994).

Dealing with the demands of caring

It may be more useful, then, in terms of intervention and service support, to examine how carers cope with an innately stressful situation and manage dementia behaviours, rather than attempt to identify social and clinical factors (which may, in any case, be unalterable) which 'cause' high levels of stress. Here, the research literature has much to offer. The broad message from various studies is that 'affective' and 'active' methods are more likely to reduce carers' stress than are avoidance or passive methods. However, as with other variables in this area, the relationships are sometimes complex (Levesque *et al.* 1995).

'Affective management' involves showing the sufferer that the carer gives 'affective support' – for example, when the carer tells the sufferer, 'you are safe with me'. These affective strategies are felt to be clinically helpful in facilitating desired behaviour in the sufferer, although there was no link between them and carers' psychological distress in Levesque *et al.'s* 1995 study. However, they were found to be associated with positive feelings about the caring role and with carers' positive affect overall (Levesque *et al.* 1995). By contrast, 'rational' management of dementia – characterised as involving the cognitive capabilities of the sufferer – for example, saying, 'try to remember' or 'do you realise what you are doing?' – was found to be associated with negative feelings about the caring role.

Matson (1994) suggests that 'tactical' coping may be, 'influential in minimizing carer stress' (p.342). This involves finding solutions to particular problems that dementia presents to carers as well as adopting more qualitative approaches, such as finding ways of meeting or balancing the needs of both carer and sufferer, and, 'showing empathy and respect for the individual, and sensitivity in interactions' (p.342). Other research hints at similar strategies being optimal. Saad *et al.* (1995), for example, found that among carers of dementia sufferers in contact with services only a few coping strategies affected carers' depression. Those associated with a reduced likelihood of depression involved being firm in directing the sufferer's behaviour and finding ways to keep him or her busy. These, perhaps, can be seen as 'problem solving' strategies and indicate 'control and mastery' over the situation. By contrast, the strategy of 'do the things you want to do and let the other things slide', which suggests a lower degree of control, was associated with carers' depression. Morris *et al.* (1988) and Orrell and Bebbington (1995) also refer to the negative effects of a perceived loss of control.

Relationships with other sources of formal and informal support
Carers repeatedly report that they appreciate formal service support, particularly home help and home care, followed by day care and aids (Wenger 1994). While dementia sufferers, and by implication their carers, appear to receive more services than other groups of disabled older people in the community (Philp *et al.* 1995), overall levels of service receipt are still low. For example, Orrell and Bebbington (1995) compared service receipt for dementia sufferers who had been admitted to a psychogeriatric assessment unit ('patients') with that of similarly affected sufferers who were living in the community (controls). They found that only 6 per cent of the patients (prior to admission) and 12 per cent of the controls (currently) had a community psychiatric nurse; 13 per cent and 30 per cent visits from a district nurse; and 31 per cent and 16 per cent a social worker. Thirty-three per cent of patients and 38 per cent of controls had received home help, with 'major' or 'full' support going to 22 per cent and 30 per cent, respectively. Given that the control sample was selected from day centre attenders and those on a waiting list, who were therefore already in contact with services, these figures probably overestimate the formal service support which sufferers and their carers generally receive.

It is not surprising, given these low levels of service receipt, to find that the carers of dementia sufferers express high levels of unmet need for formal support. However, as with the other areas considered so far in this chapter, links between what might be thought of as 'obvious' factors which would influence carers' stress and objective measures of that stress remain unequivocal. What carers report as important to them in terms of support is not always associated with lower measured levels of psychological distress or morbidity. Levin *et al.* (1983) identified home help, visits from community nurses, and day and respite care as associated with reduced stress levels in carers, and Gilhooly (1984) also pointed to the positive impact of home help and community nurse input. Other studies, however, have failed to identify a direct relationship between service receipt and stress, and Morris *et al.* (1988) in their review of the literature warn that the relationship between formal support and carers' 'burden' is a complex one.

Part of the problem in the literature, as is the case with other factors examined in this chapter, may be that of definition. So, for example, when Levesque *et al.* (1995), distinguish between different aspects of service receipt – type, frequency and carer *satisfaction* with the frequency – a more complex, but probably more useful, picture emerges. First, actual frequency of service receipt was associated with positive affect (feelings) generally, regardless of how *satisfied* or not carers were with the frequency. This, the authors suggest, may be because frequent service receipt, 'may contribute to an adequate organization of the caregiver's daily schedule and hence increase their positive affect, for example, the awareness that things are going their way' (p.352). This seems to relate, again, to the sense of 'being in control'. Second, satisfaction with frequency was associated with feelings about the caring role: the less satisfied they were the more negative carers felt about their role. Further, the more satisfied carers were also more likely to report being happy with the frequency of their social activities. These relationships may be linked: a level of service support that meets carers' subjective needs is one that is likely to allow them to engage in a desired level of social activities, while being unable to carry out desired social activities may lead to negative feelings about the caring role. Finally, Levesque *et al.* (1995) found that the number of services received, 'was irrelevant to all outcomes' (p.352).

All this points, yet again, to the importance of carers' subjective needs and perceptions; it is how they *feel* about the frequency of services, rather than the actual frequency of services, that may make them feel better or worse about their situation. This also seems to be the case with informal support for carers. There is a suggestion that it is not how much help and support carers receive from others in their informal networks that is important but how satisfied or content they are with the help offered (Gilhooly 1986; Levesque *et al.* 1995). This is a pattern found among other groups of carers, too (Parker 1990).

Levesque *et al.* (1995) showed that while the size of carers' informal networks was positively related to positive affect, frequency of support from the network was unrelated to any carer 'outcomes' (psychological distress, positive affect, positive or negative feelings about caring, or satisfaction with social activities). However, *satisfaction* with the frequency of informal support from others was positively related to carers' satisfaction with social activities. The study also demonstrated that informal support is not always an unalloyed joy; conflict with others in the informal network was related to carers' psychological distress.

Implications for supporting carers

The research reviewed here has failed to demonstrate unequivocally that mainstream services for sufferers and their carers make much difference to outcomes. Further, few specifically designed interventions appear to have had much effect (Mohide *et al.* 1990; Saad *et al.* 1995). This leaves professionals with a dilemma: if nothing makes any difference to carers, then why attempt to support them at all? As has been suggested throughout, however, it is likely that research has failed to consider this issue in a suitably complex or sophisticated way. One possibility is that the wrong outcome measures have been chosen to demonstrate effects; improvements in the quality of life of the carers may be a more realistic aim than 'curing' or reducing psychological distress (Mohide *et al.* 1990). Some have suggested that carers' emotional status may have more to do with despair than with clinically defined depression or stress, 'in that the caregivers are unable to change the outcome of their relatives' condition' (Mohide *et al.* 1990, p.452).

What, then, are the practical implications of the research reviewed above for interventions and support for carers, especially in the context of the objectives of the recent community care changes?

The general thrust of service delivery in community care in Britain over the past ten years has been to improve 'targeting' (Bebbington and Davies 1983, 1993). The reorganisation of many home help services away from domestic assistance towards personal care, for example, was done on the basis that the most efficient use of public resources could be achieved by directing services towards those who were most 'dependent'. The Audit Commission's (1986) critical report, which triggered the subsequent community care changes, claimed that more people could be better supported with the available resources if these were directed towards those with the greatest needs. The White Paper on community care which eventually followed (Department of Health 1989) underlined improved targeting of home-based services on, 'those people whose need for them is greatest' as part of its first 'key' objective (para.1.11). 'Needs-led' rather than 'service-led' approaches to supporting people were emphasised in all the practice and policy guidance which followed on the passing of the NHS and Community Care Act (1990). Support for carers was also seen as another key objective of the reforms, again with the assumption that those who are most heavily burdened should be targeted. The most recent element in the process of underlining carers' central role in the delivery of community care has been the passing of the Carers (Recognition and Services) Act (1995), which gives carers a right to assessment of their own needs.

All this, of course, implies that there is some consistent and objective way of determining need and applying services to meet it. Certainly services seem more often, 'geared to the physical needs of carers than to their emotional needs' (Williams *et al.* 1995, p.235); that is, they respond to the functional limitations of the dementia sufferer rather than to the 'poor morale' of the carers. However, as the research reviewed in this chapter suggests, in relation to dementia sufferers and their carers it may be more important to attend to carers' subjective judgements of the sufferer's limitations and the impact they perceive them to have, rather than the 'objective' level of impairment sufferers have. Applying 'objective' measures of functional limitations to sufferers or of 'burden' to carers may not identify those who are most vulnerable.

As Hadjistavropoulos *et al.* (1994) conclude, 'practitioners attempting to assess and manage caregiver burden should attend to the caregivers' perceptions of patient mood and everyday functioning' (p.308). Levesque *et al.* (1995) suggest that when carers report being particularly disturbed by the dementia sufferer's behaviour or condition, 'a possible relevant intervention would be to encourage them to express their feelings of disturbance. In doing so...professionals might help the caregiver to reconsider the meaning they assign to a stressor' (p.356). Similarly, Saad *et al.* (1995) conclude that, 'interventions which offer the opportunity to explore and therefore resolve some of the negative cognitions and difficult emotions surrounding issues of powerlessness, helplessness, grief and loss as well as providing education and more generalized positive coping strategies, would be of benefit' (p.497).

Some would perhaps recognise this type of intervention as good, old-fashioned social work! Traditional 'talking' social work would also be relevant in situations where the relationship between carer and sufferer is poor, which, as we saw above, can influence both carer stress and outcomes for the sufferer (Orrell and Bebbington 1995). Further, Philp *et al.* (1995) suggest that when carers express high levels of unmet need this may, in fact, be an indicator of stress which can be reduced without necessarily increasing service use; listening to carers may be therapeutic in itself. Unfortunately, there is a general feeling that the opportunities for social work of this sort have diminished with the community care changes and the widespread introduction of care management. Similarly, the increased emphasis on tasks in community nursing, rather than a holistic approach to the patient and his or her family, may have reduced the opportunity for such potentially helpful interactions.

Although the relationship between sufferers' disturbed behaviour and carers' stress levels is not clear, there is no doubt that carers do find this aspect of dementia a problem. Given that there are now strategies for dealing with disturbed behaviour, Hinchcliffe *et al.* (1995) recommend that professionals should 'routinely' inquire about them: 'A checklist of the most common behavioural difficulties such as sleep disturbance, repeated questions and aggressive behaviour would be easily incorporated into routine...history-taking' (p.846).

This, of course, assumes that all people suffering from dementia are referred speedily to specialist services. Unfortunately, this is not always the case, especially when onset is early (Newens, Forster and Kay, 1995; Philp *et al.* 1995). GPs are key gatekeepers to specialist and supportive services and to information, as they are often the only professionals to whom carers and sufferers have ready access. However, while their knowledge of the features of dementia may be reasonable, they nonetheless have difficulties with diagnosis and management (Brodaty *et al.* 1994). The introduction of regular assessment for people over the age of 75 may help to improve the early diagnosis of dementia and, thereby, the support which carers eventually receive.

Conclusions

The research reviewed here presents policy-makers and practitioners with a number of challenges. The increased emphasis on targeting and assessment may encourage the extended use of 'objective' criteria to decide whether or not people receive assistance – level of functional impairment and ability to carry out various self-care tasks or activities of daily living, and so on. In one sense this is a step forward if it allows the most severely disabled people to be identified accurately and supported. However, for carers of dementia sufferers (and possibly for other carers too) such approaches, by themselves, may not identify those who most need support. As we have seen, even among these very heavily involved carers, some cope better than others and it is not always those whose relatives are most severely impaired who cope less well. Thus 'objective' measures and 'cut-off points' need to be tempered with a thorough understanding of how carers actually *feel* about their situation.

Some may feel that there is an equity issue here; if one carer copes with a particularly difficult situation with a certain level of formal help, why should another not do the same? Alternatively, if one carer copes with a minimum of formal help, is it fair that a less involved carer who feels differently about the situation should get more help? As Twigg and Atkin (1994) have shown, these considerations can determine professionals' attitudes towards carers and, therefore, the support offered.

However, supporting carers who are coping less well may not always be a matter of providing more services. This is not to suggest that carers should be left otherwise unsupported; appropriate services can clearly enhance their quality of life by providing them with a break from the unremitting involvement that most of them experience and allowing them to participate in desired social activities. However, helping carers to alter their appraisal or perception of the sufferer's condition and behaviour, teaching more effective management techniques for disturbed behaviour, working with the carer and sufferer to improve their relationship, and simply allowing carers to talk may all be useful interventions which do not have major resource implications.

References

Audit Commission (1986) *Making a Reality of Community Care*. London: HMSO.

Ballard, C.G., Saad, K., Coope, B., Graham, C., Gahir, M., Wilcock,G.K. and Oyebode, F. (1995) 'The aetiology of depression in the carers of dementia sufferers.' *Journal of Affective Disorders 35*, 59–63.

Bebbington, A. and Davies, B. (1983) 'Equity and efficiency in the allocation of personal social services.' *Journal of Social Policy 12*, 3, 309–330.

Bebbington, A. and Davies, B. (1993) 'Efficient targeting of community care: the case of the home help service.' *Journal of Social Policy 22*, 3, 373–391.

Brodaty, H., Howarth, G.C., Mant, A. and Kurrle, S.E. (1994) 'General practice and dementia: a national survey of Australian GPs.' *Medical Journal of Australia 160*, 1, 10–14.

Byrne, E.A. and Cunningham, C.C. (1985) 'The effects of mentally handicapped children on families.' *Journal of Child Psychology and Psychiatry 26*, 6, 847–864.

Department of Health (1989) *Caring for People: Community Care in the Next Decade and Beyond*. Cm 849. London: HMSO.

Gilhooly, M. (1983) 'Social aspects of senile dementia.' In R. Taylor and A. Gilmore (eds) *Current Trends in Gerontology: Proceedings of the 1980 Conference of the British Society of Gerontology*. Aldershot: Gower.

Gilhooly, M. (1984) 'The impact of caregiving on caregivers: factors associated with the psychological well-being of people supporting a dementing relative in the community.' *British Journal of Medical Psychology 57*, 35–44.

Gilhooly, M. (1986) 'Senile dementia: factors associated with caregivers preference for institutional care.' *British Journal of Medical Psychology 59*, 165–171.

Gilhooly, M. and Whittick, J.E. (1989) 'Expressed emotion in caregivers of the dementing elderly.' *British Journal of Medical Psychology 62*, 265–272.

Gilleard, C.J., Watt, G. and Boyd, W.D. (1981) Problems of caring for the elderly mentally infirm at home. Paper presented at the Twelfth International Congress of Gerontology, 12-17 July, Hamburg, W. Germany.

Gilleard, C.J., Gilleard, E., Gledhill, K. and Whittick, J. (1984) 'Caring for the elderly mentally infirm at home: a survey of the supporters.' *Journal of Epidemiology and Community Health 38*, 319–325.

Hadjistavropoulos, T., Taylor, S., Tuokko, H. and Beattie, B.L. (1994) 'Neurological deficits, caregivers' perception of deficits and caregiver burden.' *Journal of the American Geriatrics Society 42*, 308–314.

Hinchcliffe, A.C., Hyman, I.L., Blizard, B. and Livingston, G. (1995) 'Behavioural complications of dementia – can they be treated?' *International Journal of Geriatric Psychiatry 10*, 839–847.

Isaacs, B., Livingstone, M. and Neville, Y. (1972) *Survival of the Unfittest: A Study of Geriatric Patients in Glasgow.* London: Routledge and Kegan Paul.

Levesque, L., Cossette, S. and Laurin, L. (1995) 'A multi-dimensional examination of the psychological and social well-being of caregivers of a demented relative.' *Research on Aging 17*, 3, 332–360.

Levin, E., Sinclair, I. and Gorbach, P. (1983) *The Supporters of Confused Elderly People at Home: Extract from the Main Report.* London: National Institute of Social Work.

Levin, E., Sinclair, I. and Gorbach, P. (1989) *Families, Services and Confusion in Old Age.* Aldershot: Avebury.

Matson, N. (1994) 'Coping, caring and stress: a study of stroke carers and carers of older confused people.' *British Journal of Clinical Psychology 33*, 333–344.

Mohide, E.A., Pringle, D.M., Streiner, D.L., Gilbert, J.R., Muir, G. and Tew, M. (1990) 'A randomized trial of family caregiver support in the home management of dementia.' *Journal of the American Geriatrics Society 38*, 446–454.

Morris, R.G., Morris, L.W. and Britton, P.G. (1988) 'Factors affecting the emotional wellbeing of the caregivers of dementia sufferers.' *British Journal of Psychiatry 153*, 147–156.

Morris, R.G., Woods, R.T., Davies, K.S. and Morris, L.W. (1991) 'Gender differences in carers of dementia studies.' *British Journal of Psychiatry 158*, (Suppl. 10), 69–74.

Newens, A.J., Forster, D.P. and Kay, D.W.K. (1995) 'Dependency and community care in presenile Alzheimer's Disease.' *British Journal of Psychiatry 166*, 777–782.

Orrell, M. and Bebbington, P. (1995) 'Social factors and psychiatric admission for senile dementia.' *International Journal of Geriatric Psychiatry 10*, 313–323.

Parker, G. (1990) *With Due Care and Attention: A Review of Research on Informal Care.* London: Family Policy Studies Centre.

Parker, G. and Lawton, D. (1994) *Different Types of Care, Different Types of Carer: Evidence from the General Household Survey.* London: HMSO.

Philp, I., McKee, K.J., Meldrum, P., Ballinger, B.R., Gilhooly, M.L.M., Gordon, D.S., Mutch, W.J. and Whittick, J.E. (1995) 'Community care for demented and non-demented elderly people: a comparison study of financial burden, service use, and unmet needs in family supporters.' *British Medical Journal 310*, 1503–1506.

Saad, K., Hartman, J., Ballard, C., Kurian, M., Graham, C. and Wilcock, G. (1995) Coping by the carers of dementia sufferers. *Age and Ageing 24*, 495-498.

Scazufca, M. and Kuipers, E. (1996) 'The impact on women of caring for the mentally ill.' In K. Abel, M. Buszewicz, S. Davison, S. Johnson and E. Staples (eds) *Planning Community Mental Health Services for Women.* London: Routledge.

Titterton, M. (1992) 'Managing threats to welfare: the search for a new paradigm of welfare.' *Journal of Social Policy 12*, 1, 1–23.

Twigg, J. and Atkin, K. (1994) *Carers Perceived: Policy and Practice in Informal Care.* Buckingham: Open University Press.

Vaughan, C.E. and Leff, J.P. (1976) 'The influence of family and social factors on the course of psychiatric illness.' *British Journal of Psychiatry 129*, 125–137.

Wenger, G. (1994) 'Dementia sufferers living at home.' *International Journal of Geriatric Psychiatry 9*, 721–733.

Williams, R., Briggs, R. and Coleman, P. (1995) 'Carer-related personality changes associated with senile dementia.' *International Journal of Geriatic Psychiatry 10*, 231–236.

Further reading

Delaney, N. and Rosenvinge, H. (1994) 'Pre-senile dementia: sufferers, carers and services.' *International Journal of Geriatric Psychiatry 10*, 597–601.

Draper, B.M., Poulos, C.J., Cole, A.M., Poulos, R.G. and Ehrlich, F. (1992) 'A comparison of caregivers for elderly stroke and dementia victims.' *Journal of the American Geriatrics Society 40*, 896–901.

Newens, A.J., Forster, D.P. and Kay, D.W.K. (1994) 'Referral patterns and diagnosis in presenile alzheimers [sic] disease: implications for general practice.' *British Journal of General Practice 44*, 405–407.

PART IV

Service Provision Issues

Chapter 9

Care Management and Dementia:
An Evaluation of the Lewisham Intensive Case Management Scheme

David Challis, Richard von Abendorff, Pamela Brown and John Chesterman

In the context of an ageing population and with the focus of recent government reforms on meeting the needs of frail people at home within increasingly tight financial constraints, services for older people with dementia will assume greater importance. This may be seen as, 'one of the greatest challenges to the development of welfare services' (Gilleard 1992, p.310). People with dementia are one of the fastest growing disabled groups in the population. This reflects the increasing number of people over 65 and the much faster growing over 85 age group where the prevalence and incidence of dementia are highest (Alzheimer's Disease Society 1994; Hofman *et al.* 1991; Jagger and Lindesay 1993; Warnes 1996). The number of people with dementia is expected to increase from 640,000 in 1991 to 900,000 by 2021 (Alzheimer's Disease Society 1994). Furthermore, between 1991 and 2011, the percentage of people with dementia living alone is estimated to increase by 59 per cent, from one-quarter to one-third of those people with dementia. These individuals make significant demands on services both in the community and hospital (Cullen *et al.* 1993). Furthermore, the increased focus on responding to the needs of carers again highlights the specific requirements of people with dementia since the carers of this client group often experience high levels of stress (Gilleard *et al.* 1984; Levin, Sinclair and Gorbach 1989), and interventions designed to prevent or reduce this are a critical element in continued dementia care in the community (Levin, Moriarty and Gorbach 1989; 1994; Lieberman and Kramer 1991; Zarit, Orr and Zarit 1985). The unpredictable and deteriorating course of the condition presents a variety of manifestations and difficulties for both clients and carers over a long period. This, coupled with the susceptibility of people with dementia to the quality of care and social environment (Kitwood 1993; Orrell and Bebbington 1995), means that providing community care for this client group presents particular challenges to services (ADSS 1994). This has led to calls for more flexible domiciliary care, both to meet the needs of isolated and confused clients (Alzheimer's Disease Society 1994) and to fit in with the needs and working hours of carers (Joshi 1995; Philp *et al.* 1995).

Services for older people with dementia and their carers

A variety of services have been identified as necessary to support people with dementia and their carers in their own homes:

- Care services including home care, home sitting, day care and respite in a residential setting (Levin *et al.* 1994). Enhanced use of professional staff in assessment, intervention and support roles, including enhanced roles for social workers (Chapman and Marshall 1993) and nurses (Greenwood and Walsh 1995), as well as specific 'psycho-educational' interventions with carers, such as individual counselling, relatives' groups, information and training (Zarit 1990).

- More intensive interventions or integration into specialist services or service systems, including community teams (Lodge and McReynolds 1984), resource centres (Donaldson and Gregson 1989; Gilleard 1992), early intervention (Keady and Nolan 1995; O'Connor *et al.* 1991), enhanced home care (Askham and Thompson 1990) and case management services (Challis 1993). Two points must be borne in mind with this categorisation. First, the distinction between these types of care is never entirely clear-cut. For example, one study outlined below, which examined the impact of a varied package of respite provision, delivered this in the context of a case management model (Lawton, Brody and Saperstein 1989). Second, important developments in psychological approaches for people with dementia themselves (Holden and Woods 1995; Kitwood and Benson 1995), such as validation, reminiscence, person-centred care and counselling approaches are not covered, since these are still rarely directly applied in people's own homes.

Sadly, too few of these services have been rigorously evaluated. When they have, the outcomes reported have been less positive in terms of delaying or preventing institutionalisation, reducing care-giver stress or improving client's quality of life (Gilhooly 1990; Gilleard 1992; Zarit 1990), particularly given the expected positive bias in reporting (Knight, Lutzky and Macofsky-Urban 1993).

This is in contrast to the positive way they are valued by carers who use them (Levin, Moriarty and Gorbach 1994). Observers have noted methodological problems (Gilhooly 1990; Knight *et al.* 1993) and a need for realism about the possible impact of services in supporting this frail client group (Gilleard 1992; Levin and Moriarty 1996). These criticisms have often focused on the service content and context, which are seen as inadequately described and often mirroring the perceived weaknesses of more traditional services: limitations in extensiveness, quantity of service (duration, intensity), quality, individuality and effectiveness of services, and the targeting of services. Connected with this has been the argument that they have often not built on the growing knowledge base of the needs and difficulties of carers and people with dementia (Gilleard 1992; Nolan, Grant and Ellis 1990).

In a series of studies considering the effectiveness of early diagnosis and provision of practical help in influencing the outcome for older people with dementia, O'Connor and colleagues (1991) examined 159 older people identified as having dementia in a two-stage community survey. Of the 159 cases, 86 individuals were referred for extra help if they or their carers wished, and the remaining 73 were provided with the usual services in the area to act as a control group. Even with provision of a wide range of help such as financial benefits, home help and respite care, permanent admission to long-term care within two years was not affected by provision of services. The authors conclude, however, that the study was conducted during the teams' formative period and greater experience as knowledge and skills developed might have permitted some individuals to remain at home for longer. Certainly some individuals were identified as 'in need' earlier than would have otherwise been the case. It appeared that older people living alone in the intervention group were admitted earlier than the control group, possibly a 'protective' response by services which was also found in a US study (Blenkner, Bloom and Neilsen 1971).

Lawton *et al.* (1989) found that a broad respite care programme embedded in a service model including case management, counselling and information for the care-givers of older people with dementia was able to maintain the older person in the community for slightly longer on average, but with no differential impact upon carers' burden or psychological well-being compared with existing services. Montgomery and Borgatta (1989) found that receipt of respite services and carer education was associated with longer community tenure. Provision of services from a specialist unit for respite and support led to significantly longer periods of time spent in the community (Donaldson and Gregson 1989). In a randomised trial of care-giver support, Mohide *et al.* (1990) found no significant impact on carer well-being, although, as in many studies, the amount of additional service offered was relatively small, being four hours per week in-home respite care. Knight *et al.* (1993) have suggested that for many studies the additional service offered is below that required to be 'an effective dose'. Zarit (1990) indicates that qualities of home care are particularly important. He suggests that reliability and degree of familial influence over the service are crucial in determining both utilisation and impact. Similar conclusions may be drawn for some UK studies. Askham and Thompson (1990) provided an evaluation of a home support scheme for dementia sufferers through the provision of additional paid carers to fill gaps in care not met by other agencies. The evaluation presented problems in terms of sample size and adequacy which made the effects of the service difficult to discern. The findings indicated no overall effects upon admissions to care homes, although some older people living alone without a carer were supported at home who would probably otherwise have entered long-term care.

Intensive care management for frail older people was examined in the Kent and Gateshead studies (Challis and Davies 1986; Challis *et al.* 1990), where case managers, working with very frail older people, controlled substantial resources and were able to create intensive, individualised support packages. Although these schemes were designed for a range of frail older people, in both cases older people with dementia were significantly more likely to remain at home than those receiving the normal services.

Levin, Sinclair and Gorbach (1989) examined the circumstances of individuals and factors associated with admission to institutional care and the effectiveness of home care. Although noting the importance of supporters' attitude to community care as crucial in determining the probability of the older person remaining at home, it was evident that provision of home help, community nursing and day care had a beneficial effect on carers' psychological well-being and that home care could reduce the likelihood of admission to care. Levin *et al.* (1994), in their study of respite services for carers, noted that an unresolved question was whether, '...more intensive community services could substantially alleviate the burden faced by those who want or have to continue to look after elderly people with moderate or severe dementia at home' (p.155).

These studies suggest at least two linked common themes. First, it is clear that the provision of the standard range of services in amounts and style of the normal kind, even if provided early, is not sufficient to have a marked impact on the probability of such individuals remaining at home or significantly to reduce carer ill-being. Second, they also suggest that it is possible that a more intensive and focused service, an 'intensive case management model' (Challis 1994), providing substantially different services both in quality and quantity, might have more impact (Levin, Sinclair and Gorbach 1989), particularly if specifically targeted upon those in need of extra support (Knight *et al.* 1993).

This chapter describes the evaluation of such a service, the Lewisham Case Management Scheme. This was an intensive case management scheme which, as such, may be contrasted to many of the services described earlier and to much care management in the UK (Department of Health 1994). The model integrates several separate aspects of intervention described earlier: the specialist domiciliary care for people with dementia (Askham and Thompson 1990), specialist mental health care (O'Connor *et al.* 1991), and intensive case management (Challis and Davies 1986; Challis *et al.* 1990).

The Lewisham Case Management Scheme: context and service model

The Lewisham Case Management Scheme was designed as one of a family of care management projects which, within the framework of an overall model, offered variation in the settings in which the service was provided and the precise target groups for whom the service was provided. Care managers, with relatively small targeted caseloads, controlled resources within an overall cost framework, so as to permit them to arrange more flexible and individualised packages of care. From Table 9.1 it can be seen that the interventions varied from the provision of social care located within a social service department for a population at risk of entry to residential care homes (Challis and Davies 1986; Challis *et al.* 1990), to location in a primary care setting where the target population was individuals at risk of hospital, nursing home or residential care placement, to the Darlington project where the service was located within a geriatric multidisciplinary team and focused upon a population eligible for placement in hospital continuing care beds (Challis *et al.* 1995).

The Lewisham scheme was established to develop a similar model of care management in a community-based service for mental health of older people. The aim of the service was to provide effective community-based long-term care which spanned the health and social service divide for older people with a diagnosis of dementia. The target population was individuals with a diagnosis of dementia, identified as having unmet needs and likely to be at risk of entry to institutional care, despite input from statutory services. Case managers with devolved budgets were responsible for providing long-term support based in the multidisciplinary team. The service setting and roles are summarised in Figure 9.1. The community-based multidisciplinary teams, which included psychiatrists, nurses, occupational therapists, social workers and psychologists with administrative support, operated an open access policy where home-based assessments were undertaken by one team member. This assessment would be taken to a case conference and a key worker approach adopted for subsequent management, drawing on the specialist skills of team members. The implications of this approach to diagnosis and treatment, and the operation of the team, are described in Coles, von Abendorff and Herzberg *et al.* (1991); Dening (1992); Collighan *et al.* (1993); MacDonald, Goddard and Poynton (1994); von Abendorff, Challis and Netten (1994); Brown, Challis and von Abendorff (1995) and Lindesay *et al.* (1996).

The case managers were located in this secondary health care setting, with a specific target population of older people with dementia, with a protected caseload of 20–25 cases, and control over a devolved budget so as to provide appropriate services. Being integrated into the mental health team and also social services employees, they had access to all the relevant health and social services resources for the care of older people with dementia.

Research design

The research was established as a quasi-experimental approach where individuals in one community team setting received care management and were compared with those in a similar community team setting without a care management service. Equivalent cases were picked up in each team by applying similar referral criteria, those with significant needs unmet by the existing services, and therefore at risk of institutionalisation. This was followed by the creation of matched groups by matching individuals on a number of key variables associated with outcome. Eligible clients and their carers were interviewed at uptake and again at 6 and 12 months. A range of indicators were used, including aspects of needs, quality of care, quality of life and well-being. These considered the perspective of the older person, carers and the assessing researcher, to capture fully any impact of the intervention. Measures used included both well-validated standard instruments, used in previous studies, or items derived from standard scales and some new measures specifically designed for this study, because of the lack of appropriate instruments for this population when the study was designed in 1988/89.

Case managers maintained structured care plans which were completed at regular intervals using a tool specifically designed for the study, the care planning and review form (CAPRE), and service utilisation and cost data were tracked through time over a 12 month period. Cost information was collected for a range of relevant parties: different agencies, older people and their carers, and society as a whole. Interviews were also undertaken with a range of key actors in the service provision process. In this chapter the focus is upon the outcomes, costs and service model for people with dementia.

The service in practice

As has been noted earlier, case managers were located within a mental health team, but with a special role focused on long-term support for people with dementia. Case managers were responsible for the assessment, co-ordination, planning and review of services for their clients through time, as summarised in Table 9.2. They did not undertake the two key tasks of case finding and screening in the ways in which they would if they were based in a front-line social services organisation. In terms of case finding, their role was to publicise the service and inform referral agents but screening and case identification would usually take place through the normal assessment processes of the mental health team. However, when the scheme specifically attracted cases in a state of crisis, the case managers on occasions undertook the initial assessment process for the team.

The case managers' assessment role would normally follow the initial diagnostic assessment by the team and focused upon assessment for specific community support packages in order to maintain the person in their own

Table 9.1 Care management studies: settings and target groups

Study	Setting	Target Population
Kent Community Care Project (Challis and Davies 1986; Davies and Challis 1986)	Social care/SSD	Residential care
Gateshead Community Care Scheme (Challis *et al.* 1988, 1990)	Social care/SSD	Residential care
Gateshead Primary Health Care Scheme (Challis *et al.* 1990)	SSD/Primary care	Hospital/Nursing home/Residential care
Darlington Community Care Project	Geriatric MDT/ SSD	Hospital long-stay care
Lewisham Case Management Scheme	Community Mental Health Team for Older People/SSD	Dementia, unmet needs, associated risk of placement

SSD   Social Services Department
MDT   Multi-disciplinary team

Shorter-Term Care

Community Team
Doctors, Nurses, Psychologist, Occupational Therapists, Social Worker
Key Workers

+

Longer-Term Care

Case Managers
Social Workers with budget
Service to dementia patients
Case Management

Figure 9.1 Lewisham Case Management Scheme: setting and roles

home, if that was the wish of the older person and their carer. Case managers would be responsible for establishing a care plan, negotiating with a range of providers of services, in particular the existing home care and other services, as well as purchasing support from outside the agency where this was most appropriate. They would also involve other mental health team members in improving the quality of their assessment and in identifying appropriate interventions. In practice it seemed that the team member most frequently used was the occupational therapist, in sharpening the quality of assessment of older people's activities and functioning. Table 9.3 shows the main services provided over one year to the matched experimental (E) and comparison (C) group cases. In general, the case management clients had significantly more home care services and more nursing contacts, we well as more diverse forms of provision. In practice it was found that despite the area in question having a relatively well-developed and extensive home care service, case managers needed to spend a considerable proportion of their budget upon purchase of home support through a range of helpers recruited by themselves and also upon services from external providers. Case managers thus spent a considerable part of their time in the recruitment, selection, training and support of local helpers to work with older people so as to be able to respond with sufficient flexibility to the needs identified. The creation of specialist additional provision reflects

Table 9.2 Case managers' roles in the care management process

Joint with Team

Case Finding	Open Access Team Context: Publicise service/inform referral agents
Screening/Case Identification	Team: Diagnostic assessment process and short-term intervention: Case managers participate in case conferences to identify cases

Case Manager Solely

Assessment	Assessment for specific community support packages by Case Manager; involve others in contribution to holistic assessment
Care Planning	Case Manager responsible for designing overall care plan
Arranging Services	Provide and negotiate services: offer direct support and continuity of involvement and indirect support through helpers
Monitoring and Review	Case Manager responsible for co-ordinating and monitoring package and review, involving others as appropriate
Closure	Placement in Residential/Nursing Home by Case Manager

the service development aspect of case management. At times this could be construed as having to in part adopt a 'provider' role, but this would be an excessively rigid interpretation since such activity has been found to be a necessary element in flexible support by care management programmes in other settings (Challis and Davies 1986; Challis *et al.* 1990; McDowell, Barniskis and Wright 1990). The helpers also contributed to the assessment of some cases.

Case managers made frequent home visits, on average more than one in each three weeks, as well as monitoring and reviewing cases both directly themselves and also, particularly regarding the client's physical health, through the paid helpers. Reviews were undertaken as and when appropriate, again involving other team members as necessary. Where community-based support was inappropriate the case manager would be responsible for organising the

Table 9.3 Patterns of service receipt: main services

Service type	E	C	E	C
	% Cases receiving services		*Service days per year alive*	
Respite care				
(overnight)				
Respite – away	32.6	34.9	6.0	10.1
Respite – in home	7.0	0	1.4	0
	% Cases receiving service		*Service days per week alive*	
Day care	41.9	42.2	0.84	0.63
	% Cases receiving service		*Hours per week alive*	
Home care and sitting				
Home care (LA)	81.4	72.1	4.0	3.6
LCMS helpers	90.7	0	7.4	0
LCMS private agency	16.3	0	0.4	0
Total home care	97.7	81.4	13.2	4.7
	% Cases receiving service		*Visits per year alive*	
Professional visits				
Community team	65.1	81.4	2.7	6.9
District nurse	55.8	58.1	15.3	10.9
Auxiliary nurse	27.9	18.6	16.0	4.6

LCMS   Lewisham Case Management Scheme
ADL   Activities of Daily Living

placement in a residential or nursing home and supporting the old person and their carers through this process.

Perhaps most significant was the case managers' role at the interface between professional intervention and care work, which can be summarised as a combination of substituting for and relieving carers, providing specialist skills and sharing the long-term responsibility. The intermeshing of social work and mental health work with care provision was manifest in a number of ways, both in response to need and in a proactive fashion. Activities included: advocating for the clients' access to services; development of the paid helper service; advising and supporting paid helpers; crisis interventions; encouraging carers to make direct contact with care providers authorised by the case manager; the introduction of care workers; and a co-ordinating role across services and agencies.

Overall, therefore, in addition to an intensive care management function, the roles of the care manager were in providing and supporting substantial levels of care resources, providing social work input, and enabling input from other services, especially the team. This role was always different from that of other team members whose function was more focused on activities of assessment, diagnosis and a shorter-term intervention (von Abendorff *et al.* 1994). Functionally, therefore, they fulfilled their aim of providing the long-term care arm to the mental health team.

Results

In the study 45 cases in the intervention group and 50 in the comparison group were assessed and followed up. From these groups 43 pairs were identified and matched by cognitive function, physical functions, disturbed behaviour, living group, level of carer stress and length of current psychiatric episode. It is upon these matched pairs that the comparisons of destinational outcome and costs are made. Due to attrition, through factors such as death, decline in health and placement in long-term care out of the area, not all would be seen at follow-up and the unmatched groups were used for the comparison of change measures. Statistical control through covariance analysis was employed for some analyses to adjust for any group difference. Given the small sample size, differences at the 10 per cent level have been reported.

Characteristics of cases and their supporters
Two-thirds of the older people lived alone and they had a mean age of 81 years. Slightly less than one-third were male. The degree of cognitive impairment as measured by the OBS score (Gurland *et al.* 1984) indicated that over 70 per cent were categorised as severely impaired. Using a composite measure of disability, the behavioural rating scale from the Clifton Assessment Procedures for the Elderly (Pattie and Gilleard 1979), 70 per cent were again categorised as of high and maximum disability. Inevitably assessment interviews with older people with cognitive impairment posed problems in about half the cases, although

Table 9.4 Destinational outcome at six-monthly intervals over two years for matched groups (n = 43)

Months after referral	At home		Placed		Dead	
	E	C	E	C	E	C
0	43	43	0	0	0	0
6	37 (86)	39 (91)	5 (12)	3 (7)	1 (2)	1 (2)
12	32 (74)	32 (74)	8 (19)	8 (19)	3 (7)	3 (7)
18	24 (56)	22 (51)	12 (28)	12 (28)	7 (16)	9 (21)
24	22 (51)	14 (33)	9 (21)	14 (33)	12 (28)	15 (35)

there were only serious difficulties in gaining intelligible views expressed by one-seventh of cases on initial interview.

In just over half of the cases the carer was a daughter or son, and one-fifth were spouses. Only 11 per cent did not have a carer. Nearly half of the carers lived in the same household or next door, and their average age was 59 years. They were in contact on average for five days per week and half of them could be deemed to be suffering marked stress or malaise (Rutter, Tizard and Whitmore 1970).

Destinational outcome and placement

Table 9.4 indicates destinational outcome at six-monthly intervals over the two year period for the pairs of matched groups. It can be seen that by the end of a year around three-quarters of each group of older people remained in their own homes, the remainder having been placed or died in similar proportions. The mortality rates of only 7 per cent in the first year and 28 per cent over the two years are very low compared with other studies of dementia, be they epidemiological studies or service populations. Thus O'Connor *et al.* (1991) found mortality rates of 29 per cent and 43 per cent, respectively, Levin, Sinclair and Gorbach (1989) found a mortality rate of 21 per cent in one year, and Levin *et al.* (1994) found a rate of 35 per cent in a study of respite services in one year.

Only in the second year is it evident that there are differences between the two groups in the rate of placement. Thus by 18 months 56 per cent of those receiving the case management service and 51 per cent of those receiving the standard community team service remained in their own homes, and at the end of two years 51 per cent of the case management group remained at home compared with only 33 per cent of those in the comparison group. Thus similar rates of placement appear to have occurred until the second year, an effect

Table 9.5 Outcomes in the first and second years after referral

Total number of people alive and at home at beginning of year (base for percentages)		Number surviving at home at end of year (%)		Number placed during year (%)		Number dying at home in year (%)	
E	C	E	C	E	C	E	C
Year 1 43	43	32(74)	32(74)	9(21)	10(23)	2(5)	2(5)
Year 2 32	32	22(69)	14(44)	7(22)	13(41)	3(9)	5(16)

Note: In comparison group 1 case placed and subsequently discharged in year 1.

Table 9.6 Change in older person needs and quality of life

	Improvement at 6 months			Improvement at 12 months		
	E	C	p	E	C	p
Satisfaction with home(C)	0.7	-0.4	<0.05	0.1	-0.1	ns
Depression(C)	1.5	0.5	ns	-0.33	0.95	ns
Client activity(I)	0.81	1.00	ns	-0.03	0.46	ns
Overall needs reduction(I)	2.9	0.6	<0.01	3.9	0.7	<0.01
Perceived change in activities and company(I)	0.91	0.30	<0.001	1.54	0.47	<0.001
ADL needs reduction (R)	2.9	0.6	<0.01	2.7	0.8	<0.05
Risk(R)	0.7	-0.1	<0.05	0.8	0.0	<0.05

Note: Sources of information: Min n = 26
       C = Older person   Max n = 73
       I = Informant
       R = Researcher

which is somewhat masked in Table 9.4 which is in effect a measure of 'prevalence' of placement.

Table 9.5 provides an indication of 'incidence' of placement when treating the two years as separate. Thus in year one there were nine placements for the case management group and ten in the comparison group, whereas in year two there were seven placements in the case management group (22% of those at home) and 13 in the comparison group (41% of those at home). Over a two year period 16 were placed in the case management group compared with 23 in the comparison group. This would appear to suggest that many of the effects of the scheme upon placement took place in the second year.

Quality of life and the needs of the older person

Table 9.6 shows the changes over 6 and 12 months, compared with initial status, on a range of indicators of quality of life and quality of care of the older person. At six months those older people receiving the case management scheme were more satisfied with their home environment. No differences were found between the groups in levels of depression (Gurland *et al.* 1984). There were no significant differences between the groups in the frequency of activities at home between the groups, as perceived by informants. On the ratings of overall need reduction and change in activities and company, there were significant gains for the case management group at both 6 and 12 months. Indicators of reduction in risk and reduction in needs specifically associated with activities of daily living, as adjudged by the research assessors, showed a significant advantage to the case management group at both 6 and 12 months, with needs and risk markedly reduced.

Carers' needs and quality of life

Table 9.7 shows a number of indicators of changes in carers' needs and quality of life for the two groups – those receiving the case management service and those receiving standard provision – at 6 and 12 months. These cover indicators of input, life strain and distress experienced by the carers. It can be seen that there was a significant reduction in the amount of total input by carers at 6 and 12 months for those receiving the case management service, and this was particularly the case for main carers evident after 12 months. In terms of overall need for client and carer and life strain for carers there was a significant reduction at 12 months on both indicators and a reduction in needs also at six months. The indicator of stress, the malaise inventory (Rutter *et al.* 1970), came close to an acceptable level of significance in favour of the experimental group at 12 months. At follow-up only one-fifth of the experimental group showed

Table 9.7 Change in carer needs and quality of life

	6 months			12 months		
	E	C	p	E	C	p
Total carer input (hours)[1]	-6.6	-1.8	<0.11	-11.2	-3.2	<0.05
Main carer input (hours)[1]	-5.9	-1.3	ns	-9.6	-1.7	<0.05
Reduced carer life strain[1,2]	0.35	0.6	ns	1.46	-0.39	<0.05
Overall needs reduction[1]	4.2	0.25	<0.001	5.1	0.6	<0.001
Malaise reduction[1]	0.6	0.4	ns	1.6	0.4	0.097
Cohabiting carers[3] Increased carer support	2.2	0.00	<0.01	1.3	-1.4	<0.01
Reduced unmet need for support	2.3	0.09	<0.05	3.0	0.1	<0.05

Note: 1 Min n = 54 Max n = 88.
2 First and second six months treated separately.
3 Min n = 12 Max n = 16.

severe symptoms, compared with 40 per cent in the comparison group. It is noteworthy that whereas just over two-thirds of carers in both groups identified a service provider to whom they could turn on referral, at follow-up all of the case management carers stated that they had someone to turn to, but still only two-thirds of the comparison group. For carers living with the older person a significantly greater level of support was provided for those receiving the case management service and also a reduction in the number of needs expressed.

In summary, although there were few expressed needs of the older person which appeared markedly different according to the indicators used, there were significant benefits which accrued to carers as a consequence of receiving the case management service, as well as reductions in the needs of the older person in the social and care domains. These positive effects occurred to the same extent for those living alone and those living with carers.

Costs

The differences in service receipt shown in Table 9.3 constitute the main differences in costs. The majority of the increased cost of case managers' cases is accounted for by home care (40 per cent of the cost differential) and by the cost of extra professional visits, including case management, and acute hospital care (around 25 per cent each). When examining only those cases still at home after one year, the increased use of hospital care accounts for one-third of the

Table 9.8 Costs to society

Costs per week	E	C	p
Total social cost	490	417	0.059
Components:			
Services	311	201	<0.01
Carers	82	111	ns
Personal expenditure	65	68	ns
Housing	32	37	ns

cost differential between the groups. When examining which sector bore this cost excess, while 70 per cent was borne by social services, 26 per cent was borne by health services.

Table 9.8 shows the costs at the most aggregated level, costs to society, for the two groups. It also shows the component parts of costs to society, namely the costs to the agencies, cost to carers, the personal expenditure of the older person and the costs of housing. It can be seen that overall there was a difference in cost, nearly significant at the 5 per cent level, between the two groups, the weekly cost of those receiving the case management service appearing to be higher. A significantly higher level of service provision was offered to older people and their carers receiving the case management service, but this in the total was to some extent offset by the lower cost incurred by carers as a result of receiving the experimental service. The balance of cost between carers and services is important as an indicator of the extent to which the scheme appeared to offer some redress in terms of provision, cost reduction and outcome to carers, one of the objectives of community care policy. One possible explanation for the lack of difference in costs is of course the lack of impact on institutionalisation in the first year, with no resultant effect upon costs. Rates of admission to nursing home care were no different between the two groups in the first year, the period in which the cost analysis is based, and cost estimates from the second year do suggest that the gap between the groups diminishes markedly as a result of the differential rate of admissions in that period.

Factors associated with variations in costs

Tables 9.9 and 9.10 show factors associated with variations in costs to the agencies per week for those individuals receiving the case management scheme and for those receiving the usual services, respectively. Underlying this ap-

Table 9.9 Average agency cost per week: care management cases

Variable type	Cost effect £	p
Outcomes		
Client - Reduced ADL needs	25.19	0.009
Carer - perceived reduction in life strain	18.50	0.05
Client characteristics		
Female sex	141.49	0.006
Depressed mood	-38.25	0.057
Single diagnosis - Alzheimer type	-100.71	0.031
Carer characteristics		
Desire for placement	79.62	0.045
Constant	50.32	0.582

Adj R^2 = 0.40   F = 5.71 p = <0.001

Table 9.10 Average agency cost per week: standard provision

Variable type	Cost effect £	p
Outcomes		
Reduced risk	29.36	0.035
Reduced depressed mood	39.10	0.007
Client characteristics		
Female sex	126.29	0.007
ADL impairment	8.26	0.05
Night disturbance	24.92	0.098
Duration of cognitive impairment	-1.23	0.009
Carer characteristics		
Reluctance to accept help	-117.19	0.049
Constant	-153.61	0.156

Adj R^2 = 0.57   F = 7.95 p = <0.001

proach was the intention to identify the determinants of variation in cost which were associated with the characteristics of the older people, their carers and the effects of services upon them, or outcomes. The underlying premise of this approach is that the ways in which costs vary are determined by the need characteristics of clients and carers and the outcomes of services such as changes in well-being over time.

In Tables 9.9 and 9.10 the material is organised into three broad domains of factors influencing costs: outcomes or change indicators, and client and carer characteristics. For both groups there is a higher cost of supporting female clients. It may be that this can be more easily understood as reduced costs for male clients due to the greater likelihood of males to have female carers who may refuse services or have services provided in smaller quantities. In the case management group older people with a single diagnosis of Alzheimer-type dementia with no other associated psychiatric diagnoses tended to be less costly. This is most likely to be explained by the fact that individuals with multiple diagnoses were more likely to exhibit a range of behaviours which are associated with higher care costs. In the comparison group, the longer the person had had a diagnosis of cognitive impairment appeared to be associated with lower costs, whereas impairment in activities of daily living and the presence of nocturnal disturbance were associated with higher costs.

There appeared to be a different effect of depressed mood in the two groups. Whereas clients with more depressed mood lowered cost in the experimental group, clients with greater reduction in depressed mood, and therefore a likely higher initial depressed mood, showed a greater cost in the comparison group. Detailed examination of these results showed that experimental clients who were depressed were either cohabiting with carers or other clients, and therefore the costs were likely to be cheaper. In contrast a number of depressed clients in the comparison group were living alone and quite a significant number of them were placed, compared with the experimental clients living alone. The differentially higher rate of placement of comparison group cases who were depressed supports the findings of Lindesay and Murphy (1989), that the Age Concern enhanced home care service appeared to eliminate this as a risk factor for placement.

In the case management group two outcome indicators entered the relationship, one a measure of reduction in needs for the older person and the other a reduction in carers' life strain. By contrast, in the comparison group, two outcomes both associated with the older persons' needs were significant, a measure of reduced risk and a measure of reduction of depressed mood. This could suggest that whereas the usual services were much more focused upon the needs of the diagnosed older person alone, the case management service was responsive both to the older person and to the broader needs of their immediate carer.

It can be seen that for the case management scheme, where the carer's attitude to placement of the older person was more positive, this was likely to increase the costs, through the association with heightened probability of placement (Levin, Sinclair and Gorbach 1989). Interestingly, in the comparison group it can be seen that where carers were somewhat reluctant to receive help costs were lower. This is again consistent with the observation that traditional services were less focused upon carers and took at face value the difficulties some carers experience in relinquishing or sharing some of the demands of care made upon them by accepting help from services.

Concluding observations

The findings of the Lewisham Case Management Scheme suggest that the impact upon older people and their carers was encouraging and contrasted markedly with the findings of other recent evaluations of specialist services for people with dementia in the UK (Askham and Thompson 1990; O'Connor *et al.* 1991). However, the evidence was less clear-cut, particularly in terms of placement, for this client group than for case management interventions for other groups of older people. There are a number of possible explanations for this. First, the nature of the service context itself was relatively resource-rich and in particular, as a consequence, the comparison group mental health service for older people was likely to provide a considerably more extensive service for older people with cognitive impairment than would be so on average throughout the UK. Hence the comparison is not between a case management service within a mental health service compared with the normal range of mental health services, but rather that of a case management service located within an enhanced mental health service compared with the presence of an enhanced mental health service. Such a context is one which is bound to minimise the kind of gain associated with the intervention. The low rate of placement in relation to other studies would seem to confirm this.

Second, it is noteworthy that the observed changes in placement rates at least took place over a longer period than the first year. Such a finding contrasts with the findings of O'Connor *et al.* (1991), who demonstrated that the presence of a specialist service *increased* institutional placement for those living alone in the second year. In the Lewisham study there was a *reduced* rate of placement both for those living alone and those cohabiting with carers, over the same longer-term outcome period. It was also evident that the presence of a new service in an area may reshape the referral behaviour of key actors. It was the case, as observed in other interventions, that the presence of the new service led to referrals of individuals whose 'care trajectory' was in a different state to that of apparently similar individuals in the comparison group. At least one possible reason for this in the early phase of the scheme appeared to be the effect of individuals referred to the service at a period of crisis, such as hospital discharge or carers past the point of benefit of enhanced support, but retained at home for the service which could only be resolved by placement, a phenomenon less likely to occur in the comparison group cases (Challis and Darton 1990; Challis and Davies 1986). Furthermore, one unintended effect of a focused service could be a more protective response to vulnerable individuals once their needs have been identified (Blenkner *et al.* 1971). This could possibly mask any other positive home maintenance effect of the scheme at the early stage.

There were significant reductions in the needs of older people and clear gains experienced by the carers of those older people as a result of the presence of the case management scheme. Importantly the impact occurred for both those living alone and with others, in contrast to other studies (Bergmann *et al.* 1978; O'Connor *et al.* 1991). The findings suggest that there are gains to be made from a more focused and intensive case management approach to this highly vulnerable group of individuals which less intensive interventions have not been able to achieve. The data suggest that such an intervention could make a cost-effective intervention in the lives of older people and their carers, particularly in situations where the carer has a desire to support the older person remaining in the community. This concurs with the logic of most studies of case management that the most effective interventions are those which are targeted on a highly specific client group in terms of the levels of need and specialised nature of the problems. The observations about the pattern of expenditure by case managers, frequently not using the existing home care services but preferring to recruit or purchase externally so as to reflect the highly idiosyncratic needs both in time and type of intervention required by this client group, do suggest that specialised rather than generic forms of home care are more likely to be successful for people with dementia.

The case management scheme – key lessons

A key characteristic of the scheme was the way in which it built upon an existing community mental health service, benefiting from the support and skills which this offered, while providing a complementary function of long-term care to the assessment, crisis work and shorter-term work of the team. The joint agency setting made possible speedy access to both health and social care resources. The case managers could effectively undertake their role, having smaller caseloads and being freed from the initial screening and assessment work. They could respond flexibly, having control over a budget for creating their own services or for use in the independent sector, as well as accessing social services resources. Their intervention was both an 'intensive' and 'clinical' case management approach (Challis 1994), and where appropriate the boundary between purchaser and provider roles could be effectively blurred to permit the needed continuity of care.

For an effective case management development there needs to be the linking of system and practice issues (Moore 1990; O'Connor 1988). At the system level, it was inevitable that there were difficulties for a small experimental project. These included limited management resources to tackle system level issues influencing practice; the small size of the team, with insufficient scale to constitute a critical mass; and the lack of information and quality assurance systems. However, despite this there were notable system level impacts as well as client level effects. Following the pilot study there has been a district-wide implementation of the case management scheme; targeting processes have been refined following the experience of the pilot study; and the paid helper service developed by the case managers which offered a wider range of social care support has been incorporated into the broader home care system and has been proposed as a model for more general home care services in mental health. Case management has also offered a distinct link for the community mental health team into long-term community-based care and has helped more clearly to delineate staff roles in this process, a development also noted in Australia (Kendig *et al.* 1992).

The essence of this service was its focus on both structure and content, placing a high priority on supporting and resourcing the clinical delivery of the service. Previous service evaluations have either focused more on content, such as providing a respite service, or on structure, such as providing an early intervention service, rather than focusing on the combination of these components and the 'implementation issues' of such services as part of a wider service system, as has been advocated for mental health services (Ford and Onyett 1996; Mechanic 1996). The role of the case manager in linking specialist mental health support together with intensive home-focused social care, and all in the context of the 'social entrepreneurial' long-term care management model, is likely to have contributed to the positive outcomes of this service model. These essential components need to be contrasted and compared with other models of provision for this client group, like the 'anticipatory care' model of resource centres advocated by Gilleard (1992) and the specialist Admiral nurse services for carers being developed in some parts of London (Greenwood and Walsh 1995). In addition, such a service can be seen as a contribution to the new culture of hope and increasing effectiveness of dementia care, oriented to client and carer needs and quality of life. The implications for practice of this kind of service model need to be related to these developments in care (Kitwood and Benson 1995).

Intensive case management must now be contrasted most clearly with the current care management arrangements. Case managers' ongoing role with cases, close work and contact with the health service and care providers, small caseloads, and the relatively large quantitative resource utilised differentiates it from generic care management arrangements (SSI 1994). This was enabled by placement of care managers in the mental health team who performed a key role in the case-finding and screening functions. And while the number of people with dementia in the community suggests that not everyone can have this kind of service, it poses questions about the way generic care management systems may need to evolve to provide more differentiated support to people which reflects their varied needs, perhaps by developing a primary/secondary distinction in social care analogous to that in health care.

Acknowledgements

The study was funded by the Department of Health, Gatsby Foundation, Lewisham Social Services and Guys and Lewisham Mental Health Trust. We are grateful to many people in Lewisham Social Services for their support and would like to thank the Guys and Lewisham Mental Health Trust for their help and support. In particular, mention must be made of the case managers, Lis Hunter, Marilyn Gross, Rita Hartigan, Dorothy Ashley and Maria Roberts, manager of the pilot project, Professor Elaine Murphy, and Professor Alistair Macdonald and our colleagues at the PSSRU.

References

Alzheimer's Disease Society (1994) *Home Alone: Living Alone with Dementia*. London: Alzheimer's Disease Society.

Askham, J. and Thompson, C. (1990) *Dementia and Home Care*. Mitcham: Age Concern.

Association of Directors of Social Services (ADSS) (1994) *Towards Community Care: ADSS Review of the First Year*. London: ADSS.

Bergmann, K., Foster, E.M., Justice, A.W. and Matthews, V. (1978) 'Management of the demented elderly patient in the community.' *British Journal of Psychiatry 132*, 441–449.

Blenkner, M., Bloom, M. and Neilsen, M. (1971) 'A research and demonstration project of protective services.' *Social Casework 52*, 483–499.

Brown, P., Challis, D. and von Abendorff, R. (1995) 'The work of a community mental health team for the elderly: referrals, caseloads, contact history and outcomes.' *International Journal of Geriatric Psychiatry 11*, 29–39.

Challis, D. (1993) 'Alternatives to long stay care.' In R. Levy, A. Burns and R. Howard (eds) *Treatment and Care in Old Age Psychiatry*. Petersfield, Hants: Wrightson Biomedical Publishing.

Challis, D. (1994) 'Factors influencing its development in the implementation of community care.' In Department of Health (ed) *Implementing Community Care*. London: Department of Health.

Challis, D. and Darton, R. (1990) 'Evaluation research and experiment in social gerontology.' In S. Peace (ed) *Researching Social Gerontology: Concepts, Methods, Issues*. London: Sage.

Challis, D. and Davies, B. (1986) *Case Management and Community Care*. Aldershot: Gower.

Challis, D., Chessum, R., Chesterman, J., Luckett, R. and Traske, K. (1988) *Community Care for the Frail Elderly: An Urban Experiment*. Cantebury: PSSRU, University of Kent.

Challis, D., Chessum, R., Chesterman, J., Luckett, R. and Traske, K. (1990) *Case Management in Social and Health Care*. Canterbury: PSSRU, University of Kent.

Challis, D., Darton, R., Johnson, L., Stone, M. and Traske, K. (1995) *Care Management and Health Care of Older People*. Aldershot: Ashgate.

Chapman, A. and Marshall, M. (1993) *Dementia: New Skills for Social Workers*. London: Jessica Kingsley Publishers.

Coles, R.J., von Abendorff, R. and Herzberg, J. (1991) 'The impact of a new community mental health team on an inner-city psychogeriatric service.' *International Journal of Geriatric Psychiatry 9*, 65–72.

Collighan, G., Macdonald, A., Herzberg, J., Philpot, M. (1993) 'An evaluation of the multidisciplinary approach to psychiatric diagnosis in elderly people.' *British Medical Journal 306*, 821–824.

Cullen, M., Blizzard, R., Livingstone, G. and Mann, A. (1993) 'The Gospel Oak project 1987–90: provisional use of community services.' *Health Trends 25*, 142–145.

Davies, B. and Challis, D. (1986) *Matching Resources to Needs in Community Care*. Aldershot: Gower.

Dening, T. (1992) 'Community psychiatry of old age: a UK perspective.' *International Journal of Geriatric Psychiatry 7*, 757–766.

Department of Health (1994) *Monitoring and Development: Care Management Special Study.* London: Department of Health.

Donaldson, C. and Gregson, B. (1989) 'Prolonging life at home: what is the cost?' *Community Medicine 11*, 200–209.

Ford, R. and Onyett, S. (1996) 'Multidisciplinary community teams: where is the wreckage?' *Journal of Mental Health 5*, 47–55.

Gilhooly, M.L.M. (1990) 'Do services delay or prevent institutionalisation of people with dementia?' Research Report 4, University of Stirling.

Gilleard, C. (1992) 'Community services for the elderly mentally infirm.' In G. Jones and B. Miesen (eds) *Care-Giving in Dementia: Research and Applications.* London: Routledge.

Gilleard, C., Belford, H., Gilleard, E., Gledhill, K. and Whittick, J. (1984) 'Emotional distress amongst the supporters of the elderly infirm.' *British Journal of Psychiatry 145*, 172–177.

Greenwood, M. and Walsh, K. (1995) 'Supporting carers in their own right.' *Journal of Dementia Care 3*, 2, 14–16.

Gurland, B., Golden, R., Teresi, J. and Challop, J. (1984) 'The SHORT-CARE: an efficient instrument for the detection of depression, dementia and disability.' *Journal of Gerontology 39*, 166–169.

Hofman, A., Rocca, W.A., Brayne, C., Bretler, M., Clarke, M., Cooper, B., Copeland, J.R.M., Dartigues, J., Da Silva Droux, A., Hagnell, O., Heeren, T., Engdal, K., Jonker, C., Lindesay, J., Lobo, A., Mann, A., Molsa, P., Morgan, K., O'Connor, D., Sulkava, R., Kay, D.W.K. and Amaducci, L. (1991) 'The prevalence of dementia in Europe: a collaborative study of 1980–1990 findings.' *International Journal of Epidemiology 20*, 736–748.

Holden, U. and Woods, R. (1995) *Positive Approaches to Dementia Care.* Edinburgh: Livingstone.

Jagger, C. and Lindesay, J. (1993) 'The epidemiology of senile dementia.' In A. Burns (ed) *Ageing and Dementia: A Methodological Approach.* London: Edward Arnold.

Joshi, H. (1995) 'The labour market and informal caring: conflict and compromise.' In I. Allen and E. Perkins (eds) *The Future of Family Care for Older People.* London: HMSO.

Keady, J. and Nolan, M. (1995) 'FADE: a strategy for action in the mild stage of dementia.' *British Journal of Nursing 4*, 22, 1335–1339.

Kendig, H., McVicar, G., Reynolds, A. and O'Brien, A. (1992) *Victorian Linkages Evaluation.* Canberra: Department of Health, Housing and Community Services.

Kitwood, T. (1993) 'Person and process in dementia.' *International Journal of Geriatric Psychiatry 8*, 541–545.

Kitwood, T. and Benson, S. (1995) *The New Culture of Dementia Care.* London: Hawker Press.

Knight, B., Lutzky, S. and Macofsky-Urban, F. (1993) 'A meta-analytic review of interventions for caregiver distress: recommendations for future research.' *Gerontologist 33*, 240–248.

Lawton, M.P., Brody, E. and Saperstein, A.R. (1989) 'A controlled study of respite services for caregivers of Alzheimer's patients.' *Gerontologist 29*, 8–16.

Levin, E. and Moriarty, J. (1996) 'Evaluating respite services.' In R. Bland (ed) *Developing Services for Older People and their Families*. London: Jessica Kingsley Publishers.

Levin, E., Sinclair, I. and Gorbach, P. (1989) *Families, Services and Confusion in Old Age*. Aldershot: Avebury.

Levin, E., Moriarty, J. and Gorbach, P. (1994) *Better for the Break*. London: HMSO.

Lieberman, M. and Kramer, J. (1991) 'Factors affecting decisions to institutionalise demented elderly.' *Gerontologist 31*, 371–374.

Lindesay, J. and Murphy, E. (1989) 'Dementia, depression and subsequent institutionalisation: the effect of home support.' *International Journal of Geriatric Psychiatry 4*, 3–9.

Lindesay, J., Herzberg, J., Collighan, G., Macdonald, A. and Philpot, M. (1996) 'Treatment decisions following assessment by multidisciplinary psychogeriatric teams.' *Psychiatric Bulletin 20*, 78–81.

Lodge, B. and MacReynolds, S. (1984) *Quadruple Support for Dementia*. London: Age Concern.

MacDonald, A., Goddard, C. and Poynton, A. (1994) 'Impact of "open-access" to specialist services: the case of community psychogeriatrics.' *International Journal of Geriatric Psychiatry 9*, 709–714.

McDowell, D., Barniskis, L. and Wright, S. (1990) 'The Wisconsin Community Options Programme: planning and packaging long term support for individuals.' In A. Howe, E. Ozanne and C. Selby-Smith (eds) *Community Care Policy and Practice: New Directions in Australia*. Victoria: Public Sector Management Institute, Monash University.

Mechanic, D. (1996) 'Emerging issues in international mental health services research.' *Psychiatric Services 47*, 371–375.

Mohide, E.A., Pringle, D.M., Streiner, D.L., Gilbert, J.R., Muir, G. and Tew, M. (1990) 'A randomised trial of family caregiver support in the home management of dementia.' *Journal of the American Geriatrics Society 38*, 446–454.

Montgomery, R. and Borgatta, E. (1989) 'The effects of alternative support strategies on family caregiving.' *Gerontologist 29*, 457–464.

Moore, S.T. (1990) 'A social work practice model of case management: the Case Management Grid.' *Social Work 35*, 444–448.

Nolan, M., Grant, G. and Ellis, M. (1990) 'Stress is in the eye of the beholder.' *Journal of Advanced Nursing 15*, 544–555.

O'Connor, G. (1988) 'Case management: system and practice.' *Social Casework 69*, 97–106.

O'Connor, D., Pollitt, P., Brook, C.P.B. and Roth, M. (1991) 'Does early intervention reduce the number of elderly people with dementia admitted to hospital?' *British Medical Journal 302*, 871–875.

Orell, M. and Bebbington, P. (1995) 'Life events and senile dementia: admission, deterioration and social environment change.' *Psychological Medicine 25*, 373–385.

Pattie, A. and Gilleard, C. (1979) *Manual of the Clifton Assessment Procedures for the Elderly*. Sevenoaks: Hodder and Stoughton.

Philp, J., McKee, K.J., Meldrum, P., Ballinger, B.R., Gilhooly, M.L.M., Gordon, D.S., Mutch, W.J. and Whittick, J.E. (1995) 'Community care for demented and non-demented elderly people: a comparison study of financial burden, service use, and unmet needs in family supporters.' *British Medical Journal 310*, 1503–1506.

Rutter, M., Tizard, J. and Whitmore, K. (1970) *Education, Health and Behaviour*. London: Longman.

SSI (Social Services Inspectorate) (1994) *Monitoring and Development: Care Management Special Study*. London: Department of Health.

von Abendorff, R., Challis, D. and Netten, A. (1994) 'Staff activity patterns in a community mental health team for older people.' *International Journal of Geriatric Psychiatry 9*, 897–906.

Warnes, A.M. (1996) 'The demography of old age.' In R. Bland (ed) *Developing Services for Older People and their Families*. London: Jessica Kingsley Publishers.

Zarit, S. (1990) 'Interventions with frail elders and their families: are they effective and why?' In M.A.P. Stephens, J.H. Crowther, S.E. Hobfall and D.L. Tennenbaum (eds) *Stress and Coping in Later-Life Families*. Washington, DC: Hemisphere.

Zarit, S., Orr, N.K. and Zarit, J.M. (1985) *The Hidden Victims of Alzheimer's Disease: Families Under Stress*. New York: New York University Press.

Further reading

Zimmer, J.G., Eggert, G.M. and Chiverton, P. (1990) 'Individual versus team case management in optimising community care for chronically ill patients with dementia.' *Journal of Aging and Health 2*, 357–372.

Chapter 10

Issues of Staffing and Therapeutic Care

Alan Gilloran and Murna Downs

Introduction

In relation to the overarching theme of the social care environment experienced by people with dementia, this chapter will be divided into two main sections. The first will focus upon social care interventions in relation to people with dementia and will cover issues of staffing by examining the following three areas:

- work satisfaction
- quality of care
- relocation and the culture of care.

The second section will examine six therapeutic interventions, grouped under two broad headings:

- reality orientation, reminiscence work and validation therapy
- group activities, expressive therapies and therapeutic touch.

In keeping with the overall aim of this volume, the chapter will endeavour to highlight the most significant contributions within the recent research literature, particularly in relation to practice issues for people working in the field of dementia care. Inevitably, however, the specific contents also reflect the research interests of the authors.

Section 1: Issues of Staffing

People with dementia receive care and support in a number of different settings and, although nearly two-thirds of this group were assessed as living in private households (63 per cent) in England in the mid-1980s, a significant minority were identified as residing in communal establishments, such as psychiatric or district general hospital wards (10 per cent), local authority residential or nursing care (10 per cent) and private residential or nursing care (9 per cent) (Schneider *et al.* 1993, p.35). Despite an overall reduction of 20 per cent in psychiatric beds in Scotland over the last 20 years, the proportion of elderly long-stay patients has increased from 45 to 66 per cent in the period from 1970 to 1988 (Scottish Home and Health Department 1990).

The emphasis throughout this chapter will therefore focus on this sizeable minority of people with dementia who receive care in residential settings. It is of course worth pointing out that many of those who are currently cared for in private households may require residential care at some point in the future. In other words these figures merely represent a snapshot in time, thereby potentially disguising the evolutionary nature of dementia care needs.

Irrespective of the precise locus of residential care, the primary underlying concern of much contemporary research lies in the quality of the care which is received by people with dementia. From a staff perspective a number of factors have been identified as influential in determining this care quality.

Work satisfaction

Philp *et al.* (1991) have compared the work satisfaction of staff in private nursing homes, geriatric wards and psychogeriatric wards and have shown that staff in psychogeriatric wards had significantly lower job satisfaction, although in relation to the item 'psychological well-being' they were interestingly ahead of the other two settings. This may perhaps be explained in relation to the work of Jones and Galliard (1983) which suggests that, contrary to popular opinion, nursing staff hold positive attitudes towards the specialty of geriatric psychiatry. Cope (1981) concludes on the basis of his study of nursing staff caring for people with dementia in various ward settings, as well as specialist units, that levels of overall dissatisfaction were high. Cope does not, however, relate the observed dissatisfaction to working with this particular type of patient; rather he concludes that work satisfaction was affected by the requirements of the organisation.

As if to reassert Cope's (1981) finding, Harper, Manasse and Newton (1992), in their study of nurses' attitudes and work satisfaction in two psychogeriatric wards, argue that, 'the organisational and managerial context of nurses' work needs to be attended to more fully in the future'. They reach this conclusion on the basis of staff comments that, 'low job satisfaction and negative work attitudes were largely the result of poor management practices and the under-resourcing of the National Health Service' (Harper *et al.* 1992, p.680).

These studies are important in that they support other work on burnout and stress (e.g. Firth *et al.* 1987; McCarthy 1985), but crucially they act to shift the emphasis away from individual inadequacies and point to structural difficulties in explanations of work dissatisfaction. Harper *et al.'s* (1992) work also concludes that job satisfaction should not be viewed as an 'undifferentiated construct' but instead it should be understood as being more complex and multi-dimensional.

In relation to work satisfaction among nursing staff, several studies have identified the important role of trained staff, particularly staff nurses. Blegen *et al.* (1992), focusing on the work satisfaction of staff nurses, examined the issue of recognition of good work by those in charge and concluded that it was more important for the nurse in charge to recognise 'outstanding performance' than merely to comment upon competent performance. Although Blegen *et al.* (1992) argue that salary increases commensurate with performance levels are a good way of demonstrating recognition, they also indicate that, 'verbal feedback to the staff nurses and written acknowledgement' are important in communicating to staff that their work has not gone unnoticed (p.63). This is an interesting argument in that it points to leadership skills as well as economic resources as influential means of encouraging job satisfaction.

In a meta-analysis of variables associated with work satisfaction among the staff nurse group, communication with supervisor and with co-workers is identified as important (Blegen 1993). Duxbury *et al.* (1984) found a significant association between head nurse 'consideration' for group members' needs and the work satisfaction levels of staff nurses. Specifically in relation to staff nurses caring for people with dementia, Gilloran *et al.* (1994) concluded that this group demonstrated lower levels of satisfaction than other direct care staff. In particular, perceptions of supervision were identified as important. For example, staff nurses were reluctant to assess their charge nurses as good leaders, with three-fifths indicating that their charge nurses did not praise them. This has led to the argument that supervision is an important determinant of job satisfaction among nursing staff caring for people with dementia (McGlew *et al.* 1991). Important too is the finding that, 'factors located in both management and the organisational structure' (Gilloran *et al.* 1994) were influential in determining the overall lower levels of job satisfaction which acts to reinforce the earlier conclusions of Cope (1981) and Harper (MIet al. (1992).

Low levels of work satisfaction obviously have important consequences for management, in that absenteeism and turnover may be adversely affected, and for staff, in that feelings of self-worth and commitment to the job may suffer. They are also likely to have an effect on people with dementia, in that an association has recently been identified between work satisfaction and the quality of care provided by staff (Robertson *et al.* 1995).

Quality of care

Through an in-depth observational study of psychogeriatric wards in four different psychiatric hospitals, Robertson *et al.* (1995) point to, 'a very strong relationship between job satisfaction and the quality of patient care' (p.575). In those wards where satisfaction levels were assessed as higher, patients were offered more choice, independence, personal attention, information and privacy, as well as a greater degree of conversation during activities such as meal times, being bathed and helped to the toilet. These activities represent occasions when patients received direct one-to-one care, or indeed at times two-to-one support, and therefore were prime opportunities for stimulation through conversation. (A full discussion of the means of measuring the quality of care may be found in Gilloran *et al.* 1993.)

Robertson *et al.* (1995) conclude by arguing that, 'management practices determine job satisfaction levels and the quality of care and that these latter two factors act to reinforce each other within the ward' (p.582). Gilloran *et al.* (1995) go on to discuss the policy and practice implications of these findings, highlighting four aspects of policy which require attention: leadership, management recognition of staff difficulties, availability of support services and pay equity. For the purposes of this review we shall focus on the first two of these recommendations.

LEADERSHIP

Good leadership entails the establishment of clear and attainable goals, as well as acting as advocate and ambassador for these ideas by leading from the front and arguing the case for proper resourcing and recognition of the importance of the work achieved. In addition Gilloran *et al.* (1995) argue that innovation, imagination and risk-taking should be incorporated into any successful strategy. Not only may such an approach subsequently benefit the people with dementia but also the staff who work with them.

Robertson *et al.* (1995) have argued that the relationship between staff work satisfaction, the quality of care received by patients and management practices is complex and in all likelihood mutually reinforcing. The quality of leadership is an integral part of this process, in that if staff can be enabled to feel good about their work then they are more likely to deliver high quality care and consequently receive further praise and recognition, which in turn reaffirms their perceptions of self-worth and commitment to the job. Encouraging and enabling leadership needs, however, to exist at both the direct care level and at the level of more senior management.

Good leadership at a face-to-face level with ward staff is important in injecting and maintaining doses of motivation. However, it is of equal significance at a greater line management distance, where support for innovative practices, for example, is a necessary ingredient. It may be possible for a dynamic ward manager to fire up his/her staff and facilitate high levels of both job satisfaction and quality of care without the concomitant support and affirmation of more senior management. However, this begs the question as to how long such an individual could plough this lone furrow?

This discussion of leadership qualities raises two straightforward issues. First, wider support from management is crucially important if good leadership is to be encouraged and allowed to flower fully. Second, dynamic, if not charismatic, leadership should be encouraged at the level of direct care staff, with the focus of attention falling on the appointment process, the assessment of leadership qualities and the availability of supportive mechanisms.

MANAGEMENT RECOGNITION OF STAFF DIFFICULTIES

Still within the area of the relationship between management and leadership, the issue of policy implementation requires attention. Particular approaches to care should be operationalised with the explicit knowledge, consent and, if possible, backing of the majority of direct care staff. The feeling of ownership is integral in terms of maintaining or enhancing job satisfaction. In the case of policy decisions which are made without the involvement of front-line staff, management should endeavour to ensure visibility of the process and to make themselves accessible for the purpose of clarifying what is intended. As anyone who has worked within an organisation will appreciate, it does not take much to foster suspicion, doubt or cynicism within the workforce which may all be rather quickly translated into dissatisfaction, demoralisation and alienation.

A further important issue for staff engaged in the care of people with dementia is training. Lardner and Nicholson (1990) have described an in-service training programme within the auspices of one particular hospital's psychogeriatric unit. Staff of all grades were enlisted to design and deliver the sessions on matters such as understanding aggression, patients' finance and attitudes to relatives. Through this process staff who had special interests could share their knowledge, which reinforced the idea that their work was both interesting and important. It also gave staff a sense of fulfilment through having addressed their peers, daunting though this often was. Such programmes of in-service training have been identified by Gilloran *et al.* (1995) as contributing to overall high levels of staff morale. Not only are such sessions personally satisfying and informative but they also crucially demonstrate a very obvious manifestation of management investment, since staff attendance and participation in the programme are built into staff work rotas.

In conclusion the identified complex relationship between work satisfaction and the quality of care, within the context of supporting people with dementia, entails movement on a number of different fronts if improvements are to be sought and achieved or indeed if current good practice is to be maintained. Probably the most important and overriding feature in attaining good quality care is the creation and implementation of a person-centred approach within an overall 'culture of dementia' (Kitwood 1993). For this to develop, and indeed flourish, a combination of supportive management and dynamic leadership is identified as a necessary ingredient.

Relocation and the culture of care

Our analysis has concentrated primarily upon dementia care received within institutional settings and we would argue that it is equally applicable to both small and large communal establishments. However, it has to be recognised that as some of the Scottish Victorian asylums close, in emulation of their southern counterparts, care for people with dementia may increasingly involve resettlement and relocation. This will entail changes for both patients and staff. Patients may become residents or tenants and nursing staff may become care or project workers. Equally staff from other backgrounds, such as social work, may find themselves increasingly working alongside health service staff. Such moves, however, involve much more than mere changes of site or indeed the renaming of jobs, in that the entire culture of care may be transformed. (For a detailed discussion of the concept of culture change within the general mental health field, see Crossan and Gilloran 1995.)

Fowler (1993) argues that the concept of culture in this context incorporates a wide array of factors such as valued qualities and characteristics, structures, systems and procedures, style, customs, beliefs and myths. It is therefore apparent that this broad conceptualisation of 'culture' is able to encapsulate both the formal and the informal aspects of social relations within an organisation.

In essence the central argument is that an approach to care which may have once appeared rational within the context of the psychiatric hospital may subsequently be perceived as out of kilter with a more community-based alternative. As well as having to face up to a potential shift in approach, staff may also be forced to engage in personal re-appraisals of their previous care work. For example, if new working practices are encouraged or instituted then what does this say about the old ways of doing things? Do staff therefore face the challenge of reinterpreting their previous best practice as having acted against the best interests of the patients (Crossan and Gilloran 1995)?

Further, cultural change may also involve having to work collaboratively with others, where health, social work and housing staff from both the statutory and the voluntary sectors may all have a part to play. The ever lurking difficulties in interprofessional co-operation in this area have recently been summarised by Soothill, Mackay and Webb (1995) and McMichael *et al.* (1995). When we enter the realm of joint working, existing power relations and established hierarchies may require to be challenged, although there is evidence from the mental health field that medical staff may still perceive themselves as occupying positions of pre-eminence even within community settings (e.g. Martin *et al.* 1995). Therefore those professional groups who have traditionally held power will have to learn to share and those who have previously been subordinate will have to participate assertively in this redistribution. As McMichael *et al.* (1995) concludes: 'we need equity in social exchange and negotiation' (p.12).

In the context of joint working, professionalism may act as an impediment, since recognised and defined areas of expertise and bodies of knowledge, which set different disciplines apart, also contain ideological and cultural perceptions which may not be so easily reconciled (Ramon 1992). In other words the simplistic notion of a variety of professionals each contributing their relevant knowledge when appropriate, ignores the potential mismatches in the fundamental understanding of a problem, the concomitant approach to care and intended or desired outcome.

For example, in dementia care if some believe in the value of risk-taking, while others prefer to opt for safety, then there is a potential difficulty. Equally, if some perceive the person with dementia as incapable of exercising choice, while others believe this to be entirely incorrect, then once again there is a problem. Finally, if attending to the physical needs of people with dementia is viewed as paramount by some but of less priority than stimulation through conversation by others, then it follows that arriving at a shared approach may prove tricky. The point is that if multidisciplinary working is to stand any chance of success then an explicit recognition of the differences in frameworks of understanding held by care staff from different backgrounds must represent an initial prerequisite. In fact to expect shared understandings is unrealistic and perhaps not even desirable, otherwise what would be the purpose and benefit of having different professional involvement?

Such a characterisation, however, implicitly assumes that there is a homogeneity of approach within particular care staff groups and across different strata within the work hierarchies of any one discipline. This may not be the case and once again it may not necessarily be desirable. On the other hand what is essential is the same explicit recognition of differences so that a process of open discussion and negotiation may be achieved.

Changes in the social care environment for people with dementia may therefore entail certain difficulties for staff who move. Interestingly McAuslane and Sperlinger (1994) found that, 'relocating residents together with their staff team appears likely to have been a major element in minimising negative relocation effects' (p.983). In contrast Collins (1994) has argued that in the area of learning disabilities staff previously employed in hospitals, but who had transferred into the community, demonstrated difficulties in breaking away from the old institutional working practices. Indeed a study into nurses' feelings after relocation from the hospital to the community indicated reactions of shock, horror and responses similar to bereavement (Massey 1991).

There is therefore a debate surrounding the best means of ensuring such relocations; in particular how best to prepare staff for the transition and how to ensure integration with other professional staff. Current research funded by the Scottish Home and Health Department, 'Changing the culture of care for people with dementia: the effect of resettlement on staff' (SHHD CSO Grant Ref K/OPR/2/2/D/265) and being conducted by the authors, is examining the process of relocation of one hospital ward for people with dementia to residential accommodation in the community.

Section 2: Social care interventions

It is well known that there is no known cause or cure for dementia. However, as with other chronic conditions, there are ways to alleviate its effect on a person's loss of independent functioning and to improve the person's quality of life.

There is no one social care intervention which will benefit all people with dementia. Approaches will have different benefits for different people at different times (Holden and Woods 1995). The intervention should be selected on an individual basis according to that person's strengths and weaknesses, abilities and interests. As such, the optimal intervention will be that which is based upon a knowledge of the whole person and not their diagnostic category (Holden and Woods 1995).

This section will discuss a variety of therapeutic interventions which challenge the therapeutic nihilism commonly found in the care of people with dementia. These include reality orientation, reminiscence work, validation therapy, group activities, expressive therapies and therapeutic touch. This is a somewhat arbitrary classification of interventions as there is considerable overlap. For example, reminiscence is often used as the basis for therapeutic group activities. However, for the purposes of discussion these approaches are dealt with separately.

This section does not discuss psychological approaches used with people with dementia, such as psychotherapy (e.g. Sinason 1992), cognitive-behaviour therapy (e.g. Thompson *et al.* 1990) or behaviour therapy (e.g. Baltes and Reisenzein 1986; Baltes, Neumann and Zank 1994; Burgio and Burgio 1986; Burgio *et al.* 1990; Engel *et al.* 1990). However, a useful overview of these approaches is provided by Holden and Woods (1995).

Reality orientation, reminiscence work and validation therapy

Reality orientation and reminiscence work are the two most commonly used psychosocial approaches when working with people with dementia (Morton and Bleathman 1991). Reality orientation can take two complementary forms: first, 24 hour individual orientation and second, reality orientation group sessions (Bleathman and Morton 1994). In 24 hour individual reality orientation every interaction is viewed as an opportunity to provide the person with dementia with verbal and visual information about what is currently happening. These visual and verbal cues are provided in order to ameliorate the disorientation which accompanies dementia (Morton and Bleathman 1991). In contrast reality orientation group sessions involve a more intensive use of individual 24 hour orientation techniques. They are generally small (three to six people with dementia) and held daily for about half an hour. While originally intended as a supplement to 24 hour individual reality orientation, in practice they have tended to replace that approach (Woods 1992).

Evaluations of reality orientation have tended to focus on orientation group sessions (Woods 1992). There is overwhelming evidence that these sessions improve verbal orientation (e.g. the person's orientation to day of the week) (Holden and Woods 1995). However, there has been some question as to the importance of this finding for the person's day-to-day life (Woods 1992). There is evidence that under some circumstances (e.g. when combined with 24 hour reality orientation) these sessions may have a positive effect on behaviour. However, this finding awaits further empirical work (Holden and Woods 1995). It is also worth stating that reality orientation group sessions increase staff's knowledge of the people with dementia who attend the group (Baines, Saxby and Ehlert 1987).

Reminiscence work with people with dementia has developed out of Butler's (1963) concept of life review for older people in general. During reminiscence work people with dementia recall past events in their lives. This work can be done on an individual (life history work) or group level (reminiscence-based activities). Cues such as music, photos and smells are used to stimulate recall (Woods *et al.* 1992).

Individual reminiscence work is more commonly called life history or autobiographical reminiscence work. This approach can be used as part of assessment and the information gathered can be incorporated into individual care plans (Gibson 1994; Woods *et al.* 1992). Life history books can be produced which tell the person's life story in words and pictures (Murphy 1994). Murphy (1994) and Gibson (1994) provide useful guides for performing life story work with people with dementia. Mills and Coleman (1994) and Mills and Walker (1994) argue that the therapeutic benefits of autobiographical reminiscence are well established for people with dementia. They argue that, 'remembering meaningful memories enhances the personhood of elderly people with dementia' (Mills and Coleman 1994, p.215). Coleman (1986) suggests that such an approach provides staff with a picture of the whole person and thus promotes individualised care.

Reminiscence-based group activities for people with dementia are extremely popular in day and residential settings (Woods *et al.* 1992). Evaluation studies suggest that reminiscence work in groups facilitates communication and brings enjoyment, but there is no evidence that it affects cognitive function (Woods 1994). It has been argued that the measure of a care approach's effectiveness should not be limited to its effect on cognition or behaviour. Rather the experience of pleasure or enjoyment should be an equally valued outcome. Gibson (1994) provides useful guidelines about conducting reminiscence-based group activities with people with dementia.

Validation therapy, as developed by Naomi Feil (Feil 1982), represents an alternative to reality orientation (Morton and Bleathman 1991). During validation therapy the person's sense of reality is affirmed regardless of its accuracy. This approach assumes that the person's behaviour and speech has an underlying meaning. As such, the listener 'validates' what is said by identifying and attending to the emotional rather than the factual content (Bleathman and Morton 1992). Like reality orientation, validation therapy can be conducted in group settings or during individual interactions. Most of the evidence about the effects of this therapy, however, is provided by anecdotal reports. Bleathman and Morton (1992) suggest that people with dementia improve in functioning during the group sessions, while Woods (1994) cautions that this approach has no demonstrable long-term effect.

Group activities, expressive therapies and therapeutic touch

The benefits of providing stimulating activities to people with dementia have been known for some time. Most of the literature on activities has centred on group activities conducted in residential and day centre settings (Mace 1987; Zgola 1987). However, activities can equally be used by carers in home settings (Teri and Logsdon 1991). The aim of therapeutic activities for people with dementia is to maintain optimal functioning and improve quality of life (Zgola 1990). Effective activities would also affect the carer's stress and frustration level (Zgola 1990).

Zgola (1990) stresses that activities for people with dementia should not be limited to traditional structured activity programmes which focus on recreation and diversionary activities, but should be broadened to include a range of daily activities. Such activities provide the person with dementia with an opportunity to experience the sense of mastery and success so severely compromised with dementia. It is important, therefore, to have a clear idea of a person's values and previous lifestyle when choosing an appropriate activity (Zgola 1990). Teri and Logsdon (1991) describe a tool which can be used to identify events and activities which are pleasant for the person with dementia.

Archibald (1993) and Bowlby (1993) provide useful guides to a variety of activities which carers can use with people with dementia. The range of activities which are possible with people with dementia are, however, being expanded with the increasing introduction of technological innovations in the multimedia field (see, for example, Maki 1994).

Expressive therapies include the use of dance, movement, visual art (Harlan 1993) and music (Aldridge 1993). Music has been shown to elicit response from people with severe dementia who do not respond to other forms of stimulation. In less impaired groups, music has been associated with improved well-being (Bright 1992). (See Holden and Woods 1995 for a review of studies on music and dementia.)

On a perhaps more individual level, aromatherapy (Henry 1993; West and Brockman 1994), relaxation (Welden and Yesavage 1982) and therapeutic touch (Holden and Woods 1995) are receiving increasing attention as therapeutic approaches to care for people with dementia.

Conclusion

The therapeutic nihilism that was once the hallmark of dementia care has been challenged in recent years with the application of therapeutic social care. Systematic research on these approaches has yet to be conducted, especially with regard to their usefulness in different settings and with different kinds of people with dementia. However, what the material in section 2 represents is a contemporary insight into the range of potential social care interventions which are increasingly becoming available. When this information is taken together with the arguments provided in the first section, then the true importance of this diverse range of social care approaches becomes apparent.

We have argued that the research evidence shows that the quality of care received by people with dementia is affected by the work satisfaction levels of care staff and that factors located in the organisational and management structures are influential. Further we have identified particular aspects within the social care environment, such as leadership and management recognition of staff difficulties, which should be carefully examined if improvements are desired or intended. We have also considered the likelihood of at least some movement by both patients/residents and nursing/care staff which may permit changes other than that of straightforward location.

We concluded our discussion of staffing issues by stating that a person-centred approach to care, which is shared by both direct care staff and management, lies at the heart of good quality care provision. Such an approach of necessity requires flexibility and a potentially individualised programme of care. Our review of current social care approaches therefore provides the tools for just such a programme. They will not, however, work on their own but instead will be dependent upon enthusiastic implementation and support in the form of the necessary resources.

Acknowledgement

The authors would like to thank Professor Mary Marshall and Mr Charlie Murphy for helpful comments on an earlier version of this chapter.

References

Aldridge, D. (1993) 'Music and Alzheimer's disease – assessment and therapy: discussion paper.' *Journal of the Royal Society of Medicine 86*, 93–95.

Archibald, D. (1993) *Activities II*. Stirling: University of Stirling Dementia Services Development Centre.

Baines, S., Saxby, P. and Ehlert, K. (1987) 'Reality orientation and reminiscence therapy: a controlled cross-over study of elderly confused people.' *British Journal of Psychiatry 151*, 222–231.

Baltes, M. and Reisenzein, R. (1986) 'The social world in long-term care institutions: psychosocial control towards dependency?' In M. Baltes and P. Baltes (eds) *The Psychology of Control and Aging*. Hillsdale, N.Y.: Earlbaum.

Baltes, M., Neuman, E. and Zank, S. (1994) 'Maintenance and rehabilitation of independence in old age: an intervention program for staff.' *Psychology and Aging 9*, 2, 179–188.

Bleathman, C. and Morton, I. (1992) 'Validation therapy: extracts from 20 groups with dementia sufferers.' *Journal of Advanced Nursing 17*, 658–666.

Bleathman, C. and Morton, I. (1994) 'Psychological treatments.' In A. Burns and R. Levy (eds) *Dementia*. London: Chapman and Hall Medical.

Blegen, M.A. 'Nurses' job satisfaction: a meta-analysis of related variables.' *Nursing Research 42*, 36–41.

Blegen, M.A., Goode, C.J., Johnson, M., Maas, M.L., McCloskey, J.C. and Moorhead, S.A. (1992) 'Recognising staff nurse job performance and achievements.' *Research in Nursing and Health 15*, 57–66.

Bowlby, C. (1993) *Therapeutic Activities for Persons Disabled by Alzheimer's Disease and Related Disorders*. Gaithersburg, MD: Aspen Publishers.

Bright, R. (1992) 'Music therapy in the management of dementia.' In G. Jones and B. Miesen (eds) *Caregiving in Dementia: Research and Applications*. London: Tavistock/Routledge.

Burgio, L. and Burgio, K. (1986) 'Behavioural gerontology: applications of behavioural methods to the problems of older adults.' *Journal of Applied Behavioural Analysis 19*, 321–328.

Burgio, L., Engel, B., Hawkins, A., McCormick, K. *et al.* (1990) 'A staff management system for maintaining improvements in continence with elderly nursing home residents.' *Journal of Applied Behavior Analysis 23*, 1, 111–118.

Butler, R. (1963) 'The life review: an interpretation of reminiscence in the aged.' *Psychiatry 26*, 65–76.

Coleman, P. (1986) *Aging and Reminiscence Processes: Social and Clinical Implications*. Chichester, NY: John Wiley and Sons.

Collins, J. (1994) *Still to be Settled: Strategies for the Resettlement of People from Mental Handicap Hospitals*. York: Joseph Rowntree Foundation.

Cope, D.E. (1981) *Organisation Development and Action Research in Hospitals*. London: Gower.

Crossan, E. and Gilloran, A. (1995) *Changing the Culture of Mental Health Care: A Literature Review for Tayside Health Board*. Edinburgh: Queen Margaret College.

Duxbury, M.L., Armstrong, G.D., Drew, D.J. and Henly, S.J. (1994) 'Head nurse leadership style with staff nurse burnout and job satisfaction in neonatal intensive care units.' *Nursing Research 33*, 97–101.

Engel, B., Burgio, L., McCormick, K., Hawkins, A. *et al.* (1990) 'Behavioural treatment of incontinence in the long-term care setting.' *Journal of the American Geriatrics Society 38*, 3, 361–363.

Feil, N. (1982) *Validation: the Feil Method.* Cleveland: Edward Feil Productions.

Firth, H., McKeown, P., McIntee, J. and Britton, P. (1987) 'Professional depression, burnout and personality in longstay nursing.' *International Journal of Nursing Studies 24*, 227–237.

Fowler, A. (1993) 'How to manage cultural change.' *Personnel Management Plus 4*, 11, 25–26.

Gibson, F. (1994) *Reminiscence and Recall.* London: Age Concern.

Gilloran, A.J., McGlew, T., McKee, K., Robertson, A. and Wight, D. (1993) 'Measuring the quality of care in psychogeriatric wards.' *Journal of Advanced Nursing 18*, 269–275.

Gilloran, A., McKinlay, A., McGlew, T., McKee, K. and Robertson, A. (1994) 'Staff nurses' work satisfaction in psychogeriatric wards.' *Journal of Advanced Nursing 20*, 997–1003.

Gilloran, A., Robertson, A., McGlew, T. and McKee, K. (1995) 'Improving work satisfaction amongst nursing staff and quality of care for elderly patients with dementia: some policy implications.' *Ageing and Society 15*, 375–391.

Harlan, J. (1993) 'The therapeutic value of art for persons with Alzheimer's disease and related disorders.' *Loss, Grief and Care 6*, 4, 99–106.

Harper, D.J., Manasse, P.R. and Newton, J.T. (1992) 'Nurses' attitudes and satisfaction in two psychogeriatric wards: their structure and correlates.' *Journal of Advanced Nursing 17*, 676–681.

Henry, J. (1993) 'Dementia – aroma groups improve the quality of life in Alzheimer's disease.' *International Journal of Aromatherapy 5*, 1, 27–29.

Holden, U. and Woods, B. (1995) *Positive Approaches to Dementia Care.* Edinburgh: Churchill Livingstone.

Jones, R.G. and Galliard, P.G. (1983) 'Exploratory study to evaluate staff attitudes towards geriatric psychiatry.' *Journal of Advanced Nursing 8*, 47–57.

Kitwood, T. (1993) 'Towards a theory of dementia care: the interpersonal process.' *Ageing and Society 13*, 51–67.

Lardner, R. and Nicholson, E. (1990) *Nurse In-Service Training in a Psychogeriatric Unit.* Stirling: University of Stirling, Dementia Services Development Centre.

Mace, N. (1987) 'Principles of activities for persons with dementia.' *Physical and Occupational Therapy in Geriatrics 5*, 3, 13–27.

Maki, O. (1994) 'Multimedia and the stimulation of old people.' Paper presented at the 10th Annual Meeting of the Alzheimer's Disease International, September, Edinburgh.

Martin, C., Allsobrook, D., Gilloran, A. and Ross, A. (1995) *Community Mental Health Resource Centre Evaluation.* Edinburgh: Scottish Health Feedback.

Massey, P. (1991) 'Institutional loss: an examination of a bereavement reaction in 22 mental health nurses leaving their institution and moving into the community.' *Journal of Advanced Nursing 16*, 573–583.

McAuslane, L. and Sperlinger, D. (1994) 'The effect of relocation on elderly people with dementia and their nursing staff.' *International Journal of Geriatric Psychiatry 9*, 981–984.

McCarthy, P. (1985) 'Burnout in psychiatric nursing.' *Journal of Advanced Nursing 10*, 305–310.

McGlew, T., Robertson, A., Gilloran, A., McKee, K., McKinlay, A. and Wight, D. (1991) 'An empirical study of job satisfaction among nurses and the quality of care received by patients in psychogeriatric wards in Scottish hospitals.' Unpublished Final Report to Scottish Home and Health Department.

McMichael, P., Grice, C., Garwood, F. and McDowall, S. (1995) *Peacemaking between the Tribes: Conflict Resolution Skills in Interdisciplinary Working in the Field of Dementia.* Stirling: University of Stirling, Dementia Services Development Centre.

Mills, M. and Coleman, P. (1994) 'Nostalgic memories in dementia: a case study.' *International Journal of Ageing and Human Development 383*, 203–219.

Mills, M. and Walker, J. (1994) 'Memory, mood and dementia: a case study.' *Journal of Aging Studies 8*, 1, 17–27.

Morton, I. and Bleathman, C. (1991) 'The effectiveness of validation therapy in dementia – a pilot study.' *International Journal of Geriatric Psychiatry 6*, 5, 327–330.

Murphy, C. (1994) *It Started with a Seashell.* Stirling: University of Stirling Dementia Services Development Centre.

Philp, I., Mutch, W., Ballinger, B. and Boyd, L. (1991) 'A comparison of care in private nursing homes, geriatric nursing homes and psychogeriatric hospitals.' *International Journal of Geriatric Psychiatry 6*, 253–258.

Ramon, S. (1992) 'Being at the receiving end of the closure process.' In S. Ramon (ed) *Psychiatric Hospital Closure.* London: Chapman and Hall.

Robertson, A., Gilloran, A., McGlew, T., McKee, K., McKinley, A. and Wight, D. (1995) 'Nurses' job satisfaction and the quality of care received by patients in psychogeriatric wards.' *International Journal of Geriatric Psychiatry 10*, 575–584.

Schneider, J., Kavanagh, S., Knapp, M., Beecham, J. and Netten, A. (1993) 'Elderly people with advanced cognitive impairment in England: resource use and costs.' *Ageing and Society 13*, 27–50.

Scottish Home and Health Department (1990) *Inpatient Data 1987 and 1988 (Mental Illness Hospitals, Psychiatric Units and Mental Handicap Hospitals).* Edinburgh: Scottish Health Service Common Services Agency.

Sinason, V. (1992) 'The man who was losing his brain.' In V. Sinason (ed) *Mental Handicap and Human Condition: New Approaches from the Tavistock.* London: Free Association Books.

Soothill, K., Mackay, L. and Webb, C. (eds) (1995) *Interprofessional Relations in Health Care.* London: Edward Arnold.

Teri, L. and Logsdon, R.G. (1991) 'Identifying pleasant activities for Alzheimer's disease patients: the pleasant events schedule.' *Gerontologist 31*, 1, 124–127.

Thompson, L.W., Wagner, B., Zeiss, A. and Gallagher, D. (1990) 'Cognitive behavioural therapy with early stage Alzheimer's patients: an exploratory view of the utility of this approach.' In E. Light and B. Lebowitz (eds) *Alzheimer's Disease Treatment and Family Stress: Directions for Research.* London: Hemisphere Publishing Corporation.

Welden, S. and Yesavage, J. (1982) 'Behavioural improvement with relaxation training in senile dementia.' *Clinical Gerontologist 1*, 45–49.

West, B. and Brockman, S. (1994) 'The calming power of aromatherapy.' *Journal of Dementia Care 2*, 2, 20–22.

Woods, B. (1992) 'What can be learned from studies on reality orientation?' In G. Jones and B. Miesen (eds) *Caregiving in Dementia: Research and Applications.* London: Tavistock/Routledge.

Woods, B. (1994) 'Management of memory impairment in older people with dementia.' *International Review of Psychiatry 6*, 2–3, 153–161.

Woods, B., Portnoy, S., Head, D. and Jones, G. (1992) 'Reminiscence and life review with persons with dementia: Which way forward?' In G. Jones and B. Miesen (eds) *Caregiving in Dementia: Research and Applications.* London: Tavistock/Routledge.

Zgola, J. (1987) *Doing Things.* London: Johns Hopkins University Press.

Zgola, J. (1990) 'Therapeutic activities.' In N. Mace (ed) *Dementia Care – Patient, Family and Community.* London: Johns Hopkins University Press.

Chapter 11

Therapeutic Design for People with Dementia

Mary Marshall

The new culture of care for people with dementia (Kitwood and Benson 1995) starts from an understanding of the fact that the functioning of people with dementia is crucially dependent on the degree of neurological damage, the previous personality and the current social and built environment. People with dementia function at very different levels with the same degree of neurological damage, so the question has to be answered about the nature of the mediating factors. This chapter looks at the impact of the built environment. Taira (1990) reminds us that the environment has the greatest effect on the person with the least capacity.

In terms of design it is usually helpful to take a disability approach rather than a pathological one because disability is something for which design can compensate. You cannot, for example, treat blindness through the design of a building but you can make it more or less easy for a blind person to function independently. The same is true of dementia, although the notion of dementia as a disability is far from well established.

Dementia as a disability is characterised by:

- impaired memory
- impaired ability to learn
- impaired ability to reason
- high levels of stress.

There are, of course, other disabilities arising from dementia in different individuals because this is a complex illness affecting different parts of the brain to different extents. Jacques (1992) provides an authoritative and readable basic text on dementia. People with dementia will also be experiencing the same sort of age-related illnesses and disabilities as any older person, although their ability to manage them may be considerably less.

The four disabilities listed above are generally experienced by most people with dementia. I want to look at how design might compensate for each of these in this chapter. First it is important to mention the people caring for the person with dementia. Their needs also have to be met by any building.

People caring for people with dementia need to feel valued by design. They also live in the buildings. This is most true of relatives at home who often live with the person with dementia. Houses that incorporate designs for dementia have to be pleasant places for the relatives too. At the moment knowledge about designing ordinary housing to meet the needs of people with dementia is in its very early stages. A scheme in Edinburgh which incorporates disorientation as a disability into its barrier-free design (Martin 1992) specifies, for example, that the doors open to give a view of the room behind. The reasons for this will become obvious later in this chapter but these features are unlikely to make a great deal of difference for relatives.

In day and long-stay care settings the needs of both friends and relatives who visit and share the care, and of the paid staff must be taken into account. A building reflects the preoccupations of those who wrote the brief and those who designed it, and it is often obvious to relatives, friends and staff that their needs were not on the agenda. This chapter will therefore include a section on designing for relatives, friends and staff.

A more positive way of saying that a building affects the preoccupations of those who wrote the brief and those who designed it is to say that a building has to be an expression of the principles of care. In a fundamental sense a building reflects the value the people responsible for it place on the people who will be using it. In some instances it is easy to see that people with dementia are seen as having less value than other groups. There is often less investment in buildings for people with dementia than, for example, people with learning disabilities.

On a more practical level the building should reflect philosophies in terms of matters such as who is it going to care for? What expectations are there about regime? What is the purpose of the care provided? Cohen and Weisman (1991) provide a useful checklist of nine therapeutic goals: ensure safety and security, support functional activity through meaningful activity, maximise awareness and orientation, provide opportunities for stimulation and change, adapt to changing needs, establish links to the healthy and familiar, provide opportunities for socialisation and protest the need for privacy. Lawton (1987), perhaps the major academic in the field of 'person–environment relations', emphasises the need for planning groups to involve architects, administrators, professionals and users. He suggests that architects should spend time with potential users to gain an understanding of their needs.

Identifying the group of people who will be living in the building is not always straightforward. People with dementia are not one homogeneous group. Assessment scales demonstrate the range of characteristics that need to be considered. The revised Elderly Persons Disability Scale (REPDS) (McCulloch 1995), for example, has seven dependency factors: nursing care, physical care, sociability, confusion, behaviour, psychiatric disorder and self-help. People with high scores on behaviour difficulties may need a building where they can see and be seen by staff, whereas people who are very confused but retain social skills may need smaller, more private areas. People in the terminal stages may have special requirements too. Coons (1991) identifies homogeneity of the population, as to needs and degrees of impairment, as a key criterion for a therapeutic milieu. Diagnosis in itself is insufficient. In the UK we are not yet very sophisticated about grouping people with shared dependencies in order to maximise the benefits of specialised buildings and staff (Marshall 1995). This has to be weighed against the disadvantages of moving people.

I am assuming for this chapter that all buildings designed for older people with and without dementia are designed to compensate for the common disabilities of old age. Valins (1988) provides a thorough and well-illustrated guide for architects and clients. Most people with dementia will be in non-specialist settings. These need to be designed to assist them. Designing for dementia will assist all users of the building in that they are generally about making a building make sense and making it easy to find your way around it.

There are ways of designing to compensate for the main disabilities experienced by people with dementia and discussion of these follow. There is a very great deal of consensus in the design literature, whether it originates in the USA: Cohen and Weisman (1991), Cohen and Day (1993), Calkins (1988), Peppard (1991), Shroyer *et al.* (1989); Scandinavia: Annerstedt *et al.* (1993) or the UK: Norman (1987), Netten (1993), Kelly (1993). Most of these authors are writing about long-stay care facilities, but many of the lessons are transferable to other buildings such as day centres and to ordinary houses. There is a dearth of good research about design features specifically since it is very hard to isolate these from all the other components of care. Much of the literature represents the accumulated experience of providers and architects. Although most of it refers to new buildings, many of the design features can to some extent be incorporated into existing buildings.

Covering design features as they compensate for the disabilities of dementia means a degree of overlap between sections, but the aim is to assist readers to understand the significance of the design of the built environment for people with dementia and to be able to think it through for themselves. Chapters like this cannot cover all design features. They are more useful if they assist in the understanding of the significance of design.

Impaired memory

People with dementia will usually forget more recent learning first. A person born in another country will tend to forget the acquired language. They will also forget first the customs and traditions of their second homeland. If we are designing a building for elderly Greek people it will need to have some of the characteristics of the homes in which they lived in the past if they are to feel that they are at home to any extent. The same applies to people who were born when buildings in the UK were different. Many people with dementia feel confused and estranged because they have no memory of living in modern buildings. If we want to compensate for this we need to design buildings which do not require recent memory. Many modern facilities look like airport hotels: smart, large and anonymous, and a totally unfamiliar environment to most people aged 75 plus.

Living with a group of other people will be a new experience for most people with dementia and one which they may have the greatest difficulty understanding. We need to ensure that the built environment is as familiar as it can be given the strangeness of the living arrangements.

People with dementia are unlikely to remember why they moved from their homes and where they are now. For most of them the place they will be able to remember is the house they lived in. If we want them to feel confident and secure we need to build small, homely units with many of the characteristics of their previous homes.

Age-appropriate furniture and fittings can be a great help. The assessment and respite unit in Stratheden hospital in Fife (Archibald 1996) is furnished from auction rooms to be as similar to the homes of elderly people as possible. It has big, old-fashioned bedroom suites with double beds and candlewick bedspreads. The ornaments are all of the 1940s and '50s. The staff believe that people who are coming in for a short stay soon feel very much at home.

One of the difficulties is providing for very mixed populations in terms of their most familiar kind of building. The homes with which they are most familiar will be very different. There are two ways of dealing with this. One is to provide local facilities which cater for a relatively homogeneous population as far as tastes and background are concerned. Another is to ensure that every resident has a room without fitted furniture which can accommodate the furniture they bring from their own homes or of the type which they would have had. They will at least feel more at home among familiar things in their own room. Relatives may have to be persuaded that their mother's old and well-worn furniture is more familiar and therefore orienting to her than a completely new smart modern suite.

Building local facilities has many advantages besides a degree of cultural homogeneity in the residents. It means that the external environment will be familiar to some extent. I met a woman with dementia who spent her day looking out on the street from a first floor landing of a very modern and clinical nursing home. It was explained to me that she had always shopped in this street and she felt very comfortable watching a familiar world go by. A local facility will also enable residents to occupy themselves in familiar places such as local post offices, hairdressers and betting shops. It will also increase the likelihood that familiar people will keep in touch. Green (1989) has provided a guide that specifically focuses on small-scale buildings that can be used to promote the development of a neighbourhood care service. He points out the possibilities for re-use or modification of existing local buildings.

More seriously, people with dementia may begin to forget their relatives and friends. They may also forget who they were and are and may experience some bewilderment and distress as a consequence. Being surrounded by familiar objects can reinforce identity: a three-dimensional life story book in a sense (Murphy 1994). This is a major part of the current approach to reality orientation (Woods 1994). Photographs can assist some people with dementia to remember relatives and friends, especially if staff use these as topics of conversation and thereby as constant reminders.

Impaired ability to learn

It is not practicable to expect people with dementia to learn to find their way, although some do to a remarkable extent. A building should be designed to make the location of essential places as obvious as possible. The best way of doing this is to ensure that all important places can be seen.

Perhaps the most important place a resident with dementia needs to get to is the WC. Not every resident will be able to get there independently but being able to see it will assist many people. This may mean having the door to the WC visible from everywhere: the dining room, the sitting room and the bedrooms. Not every resident will be able to recognise the door and some clues may help. Colour is potentially useful. However, with increasing age most people have impaired ability to perceive certain colours such as greens, blues and purples. Distinguishing between dark shades of navy, brown and black is very difficult and differentiating between blues, beiges and pinks is often impossible (Christenson 1990). Therefore if colour is to be used as a clue it needs to be in very strong contrast to its surroundings. Ferrard House (Gibson 1991), for example, has plum-coloured doors and Pepper Tree Lodge (Fleming 1991) has yellow WC doors.

Signs can be helpful. Wilkinson *et al.* (1995) found that the most effective sign for patients earlier on in their stay in the units was a picture of a WC and the word 'toilet'. Many units have meaningless modern signage and it is often placed far too high for most people with dementia. A nursing home I visited recently reckoned that by painting the door frame red and putting a sign on the door they had reduced their use of incontinence pads by 50 per cent.

Perhaps the second most important places to find are the dining room and the sitting room. They need first to be different rooms (Shroyer *et al.* 1989). If you cannot rely on the person with dementia remembering where these rooms are there are several strategies to consider. One is to ensure that all the doors are hung in such a way to allow the inside of the room to be visible. If the room is furnished in such a way that its purpose is quite clear, then sight of it may be very helpful. Glass panelled doors and even walls can help so the resident can see what lies beyond. A unit in which the location of public rooms is familiar from the past (for instance, at the front of the house) or directs the residents naturally in their direction, will reduce the need for new learning.

Finally, finding one's own room can be a challenge in many facilities even if you do not have dementia. Once you get to the right corridor the doors often look the same and require memory of a location or a number. Much more satisfactory is to avoid corridors in designing for dementia and to ensure that people can see their room door very easily. The door itself needs to have something very familiar about it so new learning is not required. This will be different for different people. A nursing home in Norway installs people's original front door where possible. This is unlikely to be realistic on any scale but the principle can be applied. Using the number of their house or, as in communities such as Shetland where houses have names not numbers, the name of their house can be helpful. Walker House in Glasgow (Bell 1992) was faced with a narrow internal corridor of identical doors: a feature they used to their own advantage by converting it into a tenement landing with old-fash-ioned paintwork, dados and gas lights. The doors have mouldings, door knockers and brass name plates. One resident has the colour, number and name plate of her own previous front door and she has no difficulty finding her room.

Light is very important. Netten (1993) found that adequate lighting made a crucial difference to the ability of people with dementia to find their way. Good lighting means that the maximum information in the environment is visible which must assist remaining learning abilities. Lighting can be used in numerous ways. It can be used therapeutically to create appropriate atmospheres. It can be used to assist residents with impaired understanding of time to understand the time of day. It is important to provide enough switches to allow staff to control individual light fittings. External light can be particularly useful in that it also provides information about the time of day and the seasons.

Impaired reasoning

People with dementia usually have an impaired ability to work out what is going on. This can make the world very bewildering for them. In design we have an obligation to make buildings make sense. The term 'legibility' is often used to refer to the quantity, quality and stability of cues in the environment (Roberts and Algase 1988). People with dementia have an impaired ability to access and appraise environmental information and may be unable to discern any meaning in some environments. Making an environment legible can be an issue of familiarity or making everything visible, as already discussed. Buildings should not require someone with dementia to have to reason. They should not, for example, have to work out where the toilets are likely to be or how to get to their bedroom. People with dementia cannot always work out that a fire door is for emergencies only. They often gravitate towards the light of the fire door only to be frustrated by their inability to open it. They are unlikely to understand why they are locked in or why certain doors are locked. There does seem to be a rule of thumb needing research, that when a person with dementia feels confined they will often struggle to get out whereas without the sense of confinement they are more relaxed. Similarly they often shake doors to cupboards that are locked but if they are open they show no interest.

Christenson (1990) introduces a very useful concept in designing for dementia: redundant cueing. She points out that sensory changes increase as we grow older. People with dementia are no exception to this. Our ability to see, hear, smell, taste and touch all change in different ways to different extents. The environment should enhance the functioning of everyone with sensory deficits by providing redundant cueing. For example, she suggests that, 'The combined input of hearing the sound of kitchen activities, smelling the aroma of food cooking, seeing and touching the table and dishes tells us that this is the dining room' (pp.3–6) Provision of multiple input compensates for losses by making the best use of remaining sensitivities. For people with dementia who experience impaired reasoning on top of sensory losses the provision of redundant cueing will increase their chance of making sense of their environment.

People with dementia may lack the ability to understand when they are at risk. Indeed this is often the reason why they are in day or long-stay accommodation. It is important to design an environment that is safe. Windows with restricted opening, thermostatic taps, radiators with safety grills on them are all routine in most dementia facilities. Doors of rooms which are not safe to enter are often best painted the colour of the walls so they are indistinguishable. People with dementia often walk a lot, for various reasons (Allan 1994) and can put themselves at risk. Gardens can be a very neglected asset. These need to be safe in the sense of having a wall or a fence, but should be designed in such a way that this does not create a sense of confinement. This can be achieved by careful planting against the wall or fence and thus concealing it, by providing distractions in the garden and by providing paths that take the person with dementia for a walk and bring them back again, ideally to a different entrance so that they feel they have been somewhere. The latter is sometimes referred to as a 'wandering path'. Zarit, Zarit and Rosenberg-Thompson (1989) found that people living in a specialist unit rarely went into the garden without a prompt or an escort. This underlines the need to provide ordinary familiar reasons for going into the garden, such as washing lines or a potting shed.

People with dementia cannot always work out what it is they are seeing. Age-related changes in vision can affect the ability to perceive depth, and people with dementia will often lack the ability to work out what they are seeing by using other information. They can mistake a change of floor covering for a step and step up or down in a hazardous fashion (Christenson 1990) and they sometimes have difficulty distinguishing where walls meet or the wall meets the floor. They sometimes mistake shadows for objects and see an obstruction where none exists. They can see reflections as ice or water and become very apprehensive with polished floors. Realistic fruit and vegetables on wallpaper and soft furnishings can be mistaken for the real thing, and care should be taken to ensure that plastic and real plants can be eaten with impunity.

Pollock (1996) in her paper on landscape and dementia warns that people with dementia will be unable to work out why it is that certain landmarks in the garden look different at different times so, if they are to be used as an aid to orientation, they need to have conspicuous bark rather than leaves unless they are evergreen.

High levels of stress

People with dementia often exhibit understandably high levels of stress and if we are to maximise their functioning we need to design buildings in such a way that this is minimised. Many of the design features already mentioned will reduce stress. Being able to see staff and to see where you want to go can reduce stress, for example. Here I want to draw attention to the need to maintain an amount of stimulation which is manageable but at a level which does not add to stress levels.

The most obvious source of potentially stressful stimulation is noise. Many places are very noisy with far more noise than can be understood by someone with dementia. Clanking trolleys, lots of people, many different activities, meaningless music and machinery such as vacuum cleaners can combine to make an environment very disabling. There is a strong argument for small scale in the controlling of noise. Hiatt (1985) states that: 'Poorly managed and designed acoustical settings can be as great a barrier to older people as steps are to a wheelchair user' (p.16). Christenson (1990) recommends acoustical ceiling tiles as well as sound-absorbing carpets and fabrics. She also suggests that earth banks, trees and large plant material outside the unit will assist in diverting and absorbing traffic sounds in urban settings.

Many older people are too hot in modern, centrally heated facilities and can become very restless as a consequence. It is very hard to meet everybody's needs as far as heat is concerned. Once again the answer may be to ensure that their own room is heated to a temperature which they find comfortable.

Providing opportunities for stress reduction is a design issue. Bathrooms are the most obvious. A bathroom can be very much more than a place to get people clean. Thoughtfully designed it can provide a warm, comfortable, sweet-smelling place for relaxation. Sadly, far too many bathrooms double as storage places for equipment and have baths which are thoroughly intimidating. There is less and less excuse for this as attractive baths come on the market, for example the new Sovereign bath by Parker, without fearsome dials and knobs. A hoist, wrongly used, can be very frightening. Better to provide a bath with a seat to raise and lower the resident comfortably.

Another sort of stress reduction is emerging in relaxation rooms which provide a quiet, comfortable space often equipped with coloured lights, soft music and attractive textures (Moffat *et al.* 1993). These clearly have a purpose in alerting staff to the benefits of stress reduction. The need for a special room to achieve this may be unnecessary (Benson 1994) once staff have appreciated the skills of stress reduction.

Finally stress can be reduced by providing familiar activities which enhance confidence and self-esteem and mitigate against the boredom very evident in many settings. A design which provides opportunities for normal domestic activities such as cooking, cleaning, hanging out the laundry and sorting out drawers will assist staff enormously. A counter kitchen, a sink near an outside door, a washing line and non-essential drawers for the 'rummagers' ought to be standard in any unit. The Alzheimer's Disease Society design guide to day centres (1992) specifically mentions what they call a 'kitchenette', in addition to the main kitchen from which people with dementia may be excluded by health and safety regulations, where clients can share in cooking activities and enjoy familiar skills, materials and smells.

Relatives, friends and staff

Like the person with dementia, friends and relatives have to feel comfortable in the building. Single bedrooms may be the place the people can talk in comfort but some relatives prefer to be in sitting rooms. Alternative sitting rooms and places where they can make a cup of tea will often be appreciated by relatives. A multipurpose room which has comfortable furniture can double as a room for counselling, private conversations and even an overnight stay if there is a sofa bed. Woods and Macmillan (1994) provide a salutary reminder that even a local homely unit may have no impact on the strain, distress and malaise in families who continue to remain in contact. They are having to cope with adjusting to the massive changes in the person being brought about by the dementia.

The domus units in London specify, as one of the aims built into their design, that there must be good facilities for staff, enabling them to function at their best (Lindesay *et al.* 1991). This is self evident but often missed in designs. Staff need space to escape, to laugh, to cry, to have a shower. They need space for meetings, training and case conferences. They need offices off the unit where they can undertake administrative chores without interruption. Facilities for staff reflect the esteem they are held in by their employers and may be a worthwhile investment in terms of staff morale.

Staff will be assisted by units which are local, reducing their travelling time and costs. They may be assisted by good child care facilities, indeed this may be one way that units can attract qualified staff in an increasingly competitive market.

Conclusion

Nothing in this chapter is unexpected to those who can empathise with people with dementia. Imagining oneself with impaired memory, learning and reasoning leads to most of the design solutions mentioned. This is a very dynamic field at present and more and more solutions will emerge as expertise increases. Particularly fruitful will be the greater understanding of the additional difficulties for people with dementia who are experiencing the usual well-documented and researched age-related changes in mobility, the senses etc.

The encouraging aspect of design for dementia is the extent of consensus in the literature. There is some divergence of view, for example on the efficacy of colour coding, but on the whole there is unanimity. Thorough research is now urgently needed to substantiate what are, on the whole, the tricks of the trade. This research is needed because, in spite of the unanimity of views, there is still much resistance to investment in design features. There is still a fundamental lack of belief in some providers in the potential for design truly to affect the functioning of people with dementia. We are prepared to invest in research in medication and in therapeutic approaches, but rarely in design which may be equally important. It is not easy research because controlled trials are impossible and it is very hard to eliminate other variables. However Benjamin and Spector (1990) have demonstrated one useful methodology (Moos and Lemke 1985) which deserves wider application.

References

Allan, K. (1994) *Wandering*. Stirling: Dementia Services Development Centre.

Alzheimer's Disease Society (1992) *A Planning and Design Guide for Community Based Day Care Centres*. London: ADS.

Annerstedt, L. *et al.* (1993) *Group Living for People with Dementia*. Stirling: Dementia Services Development Centre.

Archibald, C. (1996) *A Moveable Feast: Examples of Respite Care Provision for People with Dementia and their Carers*. Stirling: Dementia Services Development Centre.

Bell, N. (1992) *Pink Doors and Door Knockers*. Stirling: Dementia Services Development Centre.

Benjamin, L.C. and Spector, J. (1990) 'Environments for the dementing.' *International Journal of Geriatric Psychiatry 5*, 15–24.

Benson, S. (1994) 'Sniff and doze therapy.' *Journal of Dementia Care 2*, 1, 12–14.

Calkins, M.P. (1988) *Design for Dementia Planning: Environments for the Elderly and the Confused*. Maryland: National Health Publishing.

Christenson, M.A. (1990) *Aging in the Designed Environment*. New York and London: The Haworth Press.

Cohen, U. and Day, K. (1993) *Contemporary Environments for People with Dementia.* Maryland: The Johns Hopkins University Press.

Cohen, U. and Weisman, G.D. (1991) *Holding on to Home: Designing Environments for People with Dementia.* Maryland: The Johns Hopkins University Press.

Coons, D.H. (1991) *Specialised Dementia Units.* Baltimore and London: The Johns Hopkins University Press.

Fleming, R. (1991) *Issues of Assessment and Design for Longstay Care.* Stirling: Dementia Services Development Centre.

Gibson, F. (1991) *People with Dementia: The Ferrard Approach to Care.* Edinburgh: HMSO.

Green, W. (1989) *Building for the Neighbourhood Care of Elderly People with Dementia.* London: Help the Aged.

Hiatt, L.G. (1985) 'Understanding the physical environment.' *Pride Institute Journal of Long Term Care 4,* 2, 12–22.

Jacques, A. (1992) *Understanding Dementia.* (2nd Ed). Edinburgh: Churchill Livingstone.

Kelly, M. (1993) *Designing for People with Dementia in the Context of the Building Standards.* Stirling: Dementia Services Development Centre.

Kitwood, T. and Benson, S. (eds) (1995) *The New Culture of Dementia Care.* London: Hawker Publications.

Lawton, M.P. (1987) 'Strategies in planning environments for the elderly.' *Journal of Independent Living.* Fall, 1–14.

Lindesay, J., Briggs, K., Lawes, M., Macdonald, A. and Herzberg, J. (1991) 'The Domus Philosophy: a comparative evaluation of a new approach to residential care for the demented elderly.' *International Journal of Geriatric Psychiatry 6,* 10, 727–736.

Marshall, M. (1995) *A Home for Life? Profiling of People with Dementia for Longstay Care.* Longstay Care Briefing Paper No. 2. Edinburgh: Scottish Action on Dementia.

Martin, F. (1992) *Every House You'll Ever Need: A Design Guide for Barrier Free Housing.* Edinburgh: Edinvar Housing.

McCulloch, A.E. (1995) *Monklands Home and the REPDS.* Stirling: Dementia Services Development Centre.

Moffat, N., Barker, P., Garside, M. and Freeman, C. (1993) *Snoezelen: An Experience for People with Dementia.* Chesterfield: Dorset Healthcare NHS Trust.

Moos, R.H. and Lemke, S. (1985) 'Specialised living environments for older people.' In J.E. Birren and K.W. Schaie (eds) *Handbook of the Psychology of Aging.* New York: Von Nostrand Reinhold, pp. 864–889.

Murphy, C. (1994) *It Started with a Sea Shell.* Stirling: Dementia Services Development Centre.

Netten, A. (1993) *A Positive Environment.* Aldershot: Ashgate Publishing.

Norman, A. (1987) *Severe Dementia: The Provision of Long Stay Care.* London: Centre for Policy on Ageing.

Peppard, N.R. (1991) *Special Needs Dementia Units: Design, Development and Operations.* New York: Springer Publishing Company.

Pollock, A. (1996) 'Landscaping for dementia patients.' In *Design for Dementia.* Stirling: Dementia Services Development Centre.

Roberts, B.L. and Algase, D.L. (1988) 'Victims of Alzheimer's Disease and the environment.' *Nursing Clinics of North America 23,* 1, March.

Shroyer, J.L., Hutton, J.T., Gentry, M.A., Dobbs, M.N. and Ehas, J.W. (1989) 'Alzheimer's disease: strategies for designing interiors.' *American Society of Interior Designers: The ASID Report XV,* 2, June–July, p.c-5–c-7.

Taira, E.D. (1990) 'Adaptations of the physical environment to compensate for sensory changes.' In *Aging in the Designed Environment.* New York and London: The Haworth Press, p 5.

Valins, M. (1988) *Housing for Elderly People: A Guide for Architects and Clients.* London: Architectural Press.

Wilkinson, T.J., Henschke, P.J. and Handscombe, K. (1995) 'How should toilets be labelled for people with dementia?' *Australian Journal on Ageing 13,* 4, 163–165.

Woods, B. (1994) ' Reading around ... reality orientation.' *Journal of Dementia Care 2,* 2, 24–25.

Woods, R. and Macmillan, M. (1994) 'Home at last? Impact of a local "homely" unit for dementia sufferers on their relatives.' In D. Challis, B. Davies and K. Traske (eds) *Community Care: New Agendas and Challenges from the UK and Overseas.* Hants: Arena.

Zarit, S.H., Zarit, J.M. and Rosenberg-Thompson, S. (1990) 'A Special Treatment Unit for Alzheimer's Disease: Medical, behavioural and environmental features.' *Clinical Gerontologist.* London: Haworth Press.

Further reading

Fleming, R. and Bowles, J. (1987) 'Units for the confused and disturbed elderly: development, design, programming and evaluation.' *Australian Journal on Ageing 6,* 4, 25–28.

Keen, J. (1989) 'Interiors: architecture in the lives of people with dementia.' *International Journal of Geriatric Psychiatry 4,* 255–272.

Chapter 12

Dementia: A Case for Advocacy?

Anne Burton

Introduction

Over two million people will be over the age of 80 by the year 2000 in Britain (Central Statistical Office 1991, p.25). Approximately 22 per cent of them will suffer from dementia (Greengross 1986). Many will be cared for in the community, without any adequate legislative framework to help them, their carers or those professionals striving to assist them. Greengross warns that families may have to care for 15–20 years for such frail people. There is no precedent for this on our society.

The White Paper 'Caring for People' (Department of Health and Social Security 1989) sought to address the problem, heralding a new approach to service delivery through the care management approach, whereby local authorities become arrangers and purchasers of services, rather than direct providers (para.3.1.3). The emphasis is now upon assessing need and acting as a 'broker' to purchase services, simultaneously stimulating the independent sector to widen consumer choice (para.3.4.3). However, it needs to be recognised that the principle of consumer choice conflicts with the care management approach of meeting needs through externally defined criteria (Baldwin and Parker 1988). The government's hope that care management will empower users and carers (Social Services Inspectorate 1991) is additionally subverted by guidance in the same document that needs assessments must be, 'within available resources' (Stevenson and Parsloe 1993, p.65).

A further plank of the government's reforms requires local authorities to consult with users and carers in planning services. Thornton and Tozer's (1995) study of user involvement in planning the development of service provision found that the structure of consultation, essentially meeting-based, favoured active people, thus ignoring home-bound elderly users. This clearly raises questions over how representative are the views of active elderly people, and to what extent they can speak on behalf of frail, home-bound elderly people, including people with dementia.

Precisely these issues prompted a number of agencies in the 1980s to press for the establishment of advocacy schemes for older people. Age Concern in particular has suggested a Charter of Rights to Community Care for Older People, including a right to advocacy where appropriate (Age Concern 1989). Wertheimer (1993) notes that, while many older people have carers who can act in that role, almost one-third of people over the age of 75 have no one who can help them (p.3). She and others, notably Phillipson (1990), have identified a number of situations where older people would seem to be especially vulnerable, and where they consider the support of an advocate to be particularly beneficial. While they focus upon the needs of older people in general, it is apparent that the arguments apply with even greater force in the case of people with dementia.

The need for advocacy

Critical transitions and decisions

Phillipson (1990) emphasises that advocacy is particularly important in 'critical transitions', especially admissions to institutional care, in terms of raising the quality of the decision-making (p.30). For entry to private care, advocacy is considered essential to safeguard the rights of frail and vulnerable elderly people (Marshall 1986). Allen, Hogg and Peace (1992) found that few elderly people had elected to enter care, they had been offered little choice of home and they felt they had been given too little time in which to make such an important decision. By contrast, a pilot advocacy scheme has enabled many potential residents to feel in control of their situation again (Broadley 1990), by offering support to older people undergoing assessment for care.

A recent study of hospital discharges demonstrated the impact of shorter hospital stays on older people and their carers: patients felt frightened and insecure and nursing staff had insufficient time to explain events to them and their carers (Neill and Williams 1992). Advocates could help them feel more in control, as well as support carers who often come under pressure to continue caring (O'Brien 1992).

Older people in conflict situations

With the growing numbers of frail elderly people being cared for in the community, there will inevitably arise situations where their needs and their carers' needs conflict. The new legislation (The Carers' Act of April 1995) to ensure that there are separate assessments of carers' needs will not remove areas of conflict, some of which may be intransigent and rooted in the past relationship (Homer and Gilleard 1990). While it may not be possible to resolve the conflict, an advocate can ensure that there is someone to speak up for the person with dementia.

Older people from minority ethnic groups

It has often been assumed, because demand for services is low, that minority ethnic groups prefer to care for older family members themselves and have no need for supporting services. However, Brownlie (1991) has shown that dementia poses many problems for them, and that help is indeed welcomed if it is provided in a culturally sensitive way. There would seem to be a clear role here for advocates in helping to raise awareness of the special needs of minority ethnic groups.

Older people in residential/nursing care

Counsel and Care noted in 1991 that residents frequently lacked privacy and, more worryingly, that practice on restraint appeared ambiguous. Dementia sufferers would seem to be especially vulnerable because of the difficulty in monitoring their quality of life and protecting their rights. Further problems are posed by the change of ownership of homes, especially the transfer of local authority homes to the independent sector. These developments have led Counsel and Care (1992) to recommend that advocates should be appointed for such vulnerable groups with an ongoing monitoring role.

Older people and 'consumerism'

People today are expected to be active consumers, well informed about what to expect from services and ready to seek redress when expectations are not met. The Citizen's Charter (1991) is explicit in emphasising consumer rights, demand-led services and the raising of standards in public services. Under the terms of the charter, users are entitled to explicit standards, full information on choice and services and the right to redress. However, it also seems clear that consumers need to be 'active' to exercise their rights and that they need the requisite knowledge in order to make effective demands (Barker and Peck 1987).

A number of studies have cast doubt on the role of the elderly person as an 'active consumer' – rather the opposite is demonstrated. Older people 'had their needs defined for them' and carers' needs were often unrecognised (Marsh and Fisher 1992). Demand was rationed by practitioners withholding information on criteria for services (Ellis 1993) and choice was often negative rather than positive, with users refusing services that were unsatisfactory and complaining being seen as 'the last resort' (Allen *et al.* 1992, p.325). Although the new community care arrangements have resulted in more flexible services, offering greater intensity of support, users and carers felt these changes were still relatively marginal (Henwood 1995).

McGlone's study of disability in Britain (1992) charts the growing financial divide among pensioners. Whereas 50 per cent of pensioners live on the edge of poverty, a growing number now have occupational pensions and significant wealth. The choice of care therefore, 'will largely be the prerogative of those who can pay' (p.42). The model of welfare pluralism had earlier been criticised by Mishra (1990) as eroding social justice, since there are inequities in the ability to purchase care and exercise choice. Dementia sufferers, who occupy a devalued status in society, are likely to be at a particular disadvantage, especially if they have no protective family (Fennell, Phillipson and Evers 1991).

The mixed economy of care, with resultant care packages composed of a combination of services from the statutory, voluntary and private sectors, will increasingly become the norm for the future. Although service delivery should therefore become more flexible and responsive, it could well be experienced by users, and in particular dementia sufferers, as both confusing and fragmented.

Rights and entitlements in community care
Despite the obvious inequalities noted above, it could be argued that the NHS and Community Care Act (1990) has enhanced the rights of older people and their carers, since under Section 47(1) there is a right to an assessment, 'where it appears to a local authority that any person for whom they may provide...community care services may be in need of any such services'. The needs assessment then establishes eligibility for services. However, assessment is an imperfect science, and even experienced practitioners disagree on what constitutes a 'need' (Clark 1996, p.159).

This legislation has been attacked as a retreat from a rights-based approach by Doyle and Harding (1992) and Bynoe (1993) on the grounds that it does not confer entitlement. It therefore differs significantly from the Disabled Persons Act (1986), which imposed a duty upon local authorities to assess the needs of a disabled person, and the care-planning process itself lacks a clear underpinning framework of rights.

Thus far we have looked at the potential advocacy needs of older people in general and only touched upon the particular problems of people with dementia. Since many of the problems hinge upon their capacity for decision-making, this is discussed in more detail in the following section.

Decision-making with adults with mental impairment

The practitioners in Stevenson and Parsloe's study of community care (1993) experienced great difficulties in deciding at what point a dementia sufferer has lost the capacity to exercise autonomy. In legal terms, every adult is presumed to have capacity until proved otherwise (English Law Commission 1991). Furthermore, capacity is relative both to the person's ability and to the decision under contemplation. In essence the person concerned must at the time under-stand in broad terms what they are doing and the effects of their actions. The point made is that legal capacity depends upon 'understanding rather than wisdom' (p.20), so that the quality of the decision-making is irrelevant. This raises awkward questions as to the person's real understanding of the issues and possible alternatives, their vulnerability to pressure or exploitation from others, and who should intervene if there are signs of neglect or abuse, or make significant decisions, such as entering residential care (Carson 1991).

The deficiencies of current legislation in respect of decision-making and dementia have been well documented (Scottish Action on Dementia 1988). The use of guardianship under the Mental Health (Scotland) Act (1984) to enhance decision-making in respect of adults with mental impairment is deemed insuf-ficiently flexible to cope with the differing needs of mentally disabled adults in the community (Moore *et al.* 1992). It has been used increasingly with dementia sufferers, but mostly in respect of admission to residential care, which is contrary to the spirit of the legislation (McCreadie 1989). Whereas guardians take powers to decide 'in best interests' – a paternalistic approach – advocates seek to learn what their partners' wishes are and then facilitate them – an empowerment model.

Two standards are discerned in decision-making for adults with mental impairment, which can be characterised as: (1) the 'best interests' approach and (2) the 'substituted judgement' approach (Penhale 1991). The first seems to have its origins in legislation concerned with children, and tends to be used in situations where the individual is considered never to have been capable of making competent decisions. It is therefore a paternalistic approach and, in seeking to minimise risk, could appear restrictive.

The 'substituted judgement' approach, on the other hand, seeks to preserve autonomy by referring to the known values and beliefs of the person when competent (Law Society 1989). This approach is the one most likely to be utilised by advocates working with adults who lack 'capacity' but is not, however, without difficulty. It may be difficult to establish what the person's views were, especially if there are no informants available; carers may present a distorted view in furtherance of their own interests; there may not be sufficient time to ascertain the necessary information and the person's known views could result in a decision harmful to them.

Dworkin (1986) questions the extent to which autonomy should be preserved. How far, he asks, do people with dementia have a right to make decisions for themselves that others would deem not in their best interests? He asserts that dementia sufferers should be considered as people who have been competent in the past, and whose dementia, 'has occurred in the course of a longer life whose length must be considered in any decision about what rights he has...' (pp.9–10). Dworkin's view is that where, as a consequence of their degree of mental impairment, a person's decision-making shows no coherence or the decisions are, 'radically discontinuous with the known values of his previous life', then they have lost the right to have any decision respected, 'just out of concern for their autonomy' (p.9). They do, however, have the right to beneficence, i.e. the right that decisions be made 'in his/her best interests' (Gilhooly 1992, p.27).

Decision-making with adults who lack competence is complex and difficult for practitioners and advocates alike. The decision-making process may be the focus for conflicting perspectives between professionals, between professionals and carers or between professionals and members of the community. In such situations there seems a clear role for an advocate, adopting a more independent stance, to support the dementia sufferer and to enable their voice to be heard.

The development of the advocacy movement

Advocacy means 'pleading for, or supporting' (OED definition) and first sprang up in the USA in the mid-1960s, as a response to the anxieties of parents of disabled children over who would support them after their parents' death. It has since spread to encompass other client groups and it was intended to be, 'a strategy of optimising the likelihood that an impaired person would be protected if and when there was no family that could or would do it' (Wolfensberger 1983, p.3). Advocates are described as ordinary people who partner another person, 'who risks social exclusion...because of a handicap' and who represent that person's interests as if they were the advocate's own (O'Brien 1984, p.33).

Much of the development of the advocacy movement in Britain and in the USA has been in the field of learning disabilities. Advocacy had its origins in normalisation theory, which sought to create valued roles for people at risk of exclusion or devaluation by the community (Wolfensberger 1977), and helped to shape services for people with learning disabilities moving from institutional care into the community. It was the starting point for citizen advocacy and self-advocacy (Tyne 1992).

In Britain in 1981 the UK Advocacy Alliance (now known as National Citizen Advocacy) was established to focus on people with learning disabilities in hospital. Hospital staff were initially hostile to advocates (Rankin 1989), but from these beginnings a number of advocacy schemes became established, working with, in the main, people with learning disabilities or mental health problems. Crawley (1988) has documented how advocates attempted with some success to shape service provision into more responsive patterns of delivery.

Advocacy with older people also originated in the USA, where the Older Americans Act (1978) mandated states to set up a Long Term Care Ombudsman Program, in the context of public disquiet over conditions in private nursing homes. The ombudsman programme successfully fought to secure statutory oversight of nursing home provision and, whilst resulting in an increase in complaints about the quality of care, it also led to an improvement in the standards of care (Californian Department of Aging 1990).

In Britain a growing number of advocacy schemes also offer advocacy services to older people, including dementia sufferers, many under the aegis of Age Concern. MIND has also begun to develop advocacy for older people with mental health problems, including dementia. Some projects offer advocacy to older people in the community, whereas other projects offer a service to older people in care. This may encompass advocacy for residents in local authority homes undergoing a change of ownership (see, for example, Ivers 1994), or advocacy for older people in long-term hospital care (Age Concern Scotland 1995).

Only a few projects thus far have a more specific focus on dementia. Half a dozen projects (all in Scotland) have a specific focus on advocacy with dementia sufferers, three offering one-to-one advocacy for the person with dementia, and one aiming to empower carers as advocates. One of the projects offers advocacy specifically for dementia sufferers in long-term hospital care, while another offers support to people in residential care. Finally there are two legal advocacy projects (both also in Scotland), which are sister projects offering assistance to people with mental impairment with any legal problems they may have. (Details of some of these projects are held by the Dementia Services Development Centre, University of Stirling.)

Models of advocacy and dementia

Brandon (1995) asserts that though there are many different forms of advocacy, there are only three basic kinds: self-advocacy, paid/professional advocacy and unpaid/amateur advocacy.

Self-advocacy

Self-advocacy is often described as speaking up for oneself and has particularly evolved in the field of learning disabilities and mental health in the form of collective self-advocacy. This is thought by O'Hagan to be the most empowering form of advocacy, since it helps people, 'to discover and use their own competence' (p.73). Age Concern has recently encouraged its development with older people, though not with a specific focus upon those suffering from dementia. In the latter group self-advocacy would require early diagnosis and referral, something that GPs have been reluctant to undertake (National Consumer Council 1990).

Paid/professional advocacy

Paid/professional advocacy can encompass legal advocacy, which often involves legal advice and a representation service to users. Many national organisations, e.g. MIND and MENCAP, offer such a service, and two legal services projects have developed through Mental Illness Specific Grant funding.

Also, a number of advocacy projects employ paid advocates (usually professionals), in addition to recruiting volunteer advocates, as they may offer more than one form of advocacy – for example, short-term or crisis advocacy, as well as long-term partnerships. Indeed Dunning (1995) considers that the form of advocacy may need to change to fit individuals' changed circumstances. This is particularly the case in dementia, where the progression of the disease will inevitably bring different problems in its train. Initial short-term advocacy to assist with, for example, problems of financial management, may need to develop into a longer-term partnership as the person's capacity for organising their affairs decreases, because of the need to facilitate planning for the person's future care.

Other professionals, especially hospital staff, often see themselves as the advocates for their patients (Ivers 1994; Rankin 1989). Whilst Brandon accepts that professionals have a legitimate advocacy role, which is reinforced by the dearth of 'pure' advocates, Herr (1989), however, cautions that there is an enormous temptation for professionals to be paternalistic.

Unpaid/amateur advocacy

Citizen advocacy has a long history and has its roots in the USA In essence a citizen advocate is unpaid, represents the interests of their partner as if they were their own, and is completely loyal to that partner. The relationship is a long-term one, and for that reason may not be entirely suitable to dementia, which is a deteriorating condition and could lead to situations where it is no longer clear whether a dementia sufferer is able to consent to the activities of the advocate. The risk of exploitation is therefore a real one and raises serious issues regarding the overseeing of their activities.

On the other hand, it can be argued that the length of the partnership will develop trust and, further, that knowledge of the needs and wishes of the person with dementia gained when the person was more able, will be sufficient to overcome these difficulties. Advocacy in the latter stages of dementia would therefore be enhanced by the partnership formed in the earlier stages.

The category also encompasses families as advocates. Whether families can satisfactorily act as advocates on behalf of their relatives with dementia depends on the quality of the relationship. As Brandon (1995) comments: 'Some families can be a source of oppression...' (p.49). In fact, Buchanan and Brock (1986) advise that families should not be placed in the role of decision makers as serious conflicts of interest could arise and both the Law Society (1989) and Scottish Action on Dementia (1992) recommend that advocates should be independent both of families and service providers.

A study of advocacy in action

Advocacy with dementia sufferers, however, is a new field where relatively little is known. In 1993-94 the author carried out a small but illustrative study based upon ten dementia sufferers, who had been referred to a new project offering independent one-to-one advocacy with people with dementia and employing paid advocates (Burton 1994). The aim was to clarify the impact of advocacy upon dementia sufferers and carers, as well as upon people making referral to the project. It sought to identify how advocates ensured that dementia sufferers participate in decision-making; what approaches were used; how they resolved any conflict between a dementia sufferer's expressed wishes and what they apparently need; and whether peoples' expectations of the project were met.

The study

The research was carried out by means of a structured interview with the advocate and the people who had made referral to the project over a six month time scale, together with carers and other professionals who played a significant role in each case. In all, 28 respondents were interviewed. It had also been hoped to interview the dementia sufferers referred to the project, but a pilot study revealed their level of impairment to be too severe for any useful information to be elicited. Only four of the clients had carers, and one of these was assessed as unsupportive by the referring practitioner. None was from a minority ethnic group.

Many of the clients were referred because they were faced with fairly critical decision-making over their future care and lacked anyone to speak up for them. Three clients were also at the centre of conflict between professionals over their care needs, necessitating the independent perspective of an advocate, and one client was thought to be the subject of financial abuse and needed help to express her views in attempting to resolve the difficulties. One carer requested help in her role as an advocate for her mother.

Outcomes of advocacy

Over 80 per cent of the respondents interviewed felt that the advocate had been effective in her interventions. The key areas of effectiveness were the following:

CLIENT PARTICIPATION

All of the practitioners who referred to the project indicated great satisfaction with the advocate because they felt she had been instrumental in ensuring their clients' wishes were both heard and respected. They especially appreciated her spending time with their clients to discern their preferences while they grappled with their new roles under the community care legislation, which they considered to be complex and time-consuming.

In general the social workers interviewed supported a participatory model of decision-making. Hospital nursing staff, by contrast, especially those not versed in the care of dementia sufferers, were much more likely to adopt a paternalistic stance and much less willing to involve dementia sufferers in decision-making. There seemed therefore to be something of a philosophical divide between health and social work staff which was detrimental to multidisciplinary working – some joint training in this difficult area may be mutually beneficial, which advocates would seem well placed to facilitate.

ENSURING RESOURCES WERE APPROPRIATE TO NEED

This was a problem area in at least four of the ten cases in the study. Arguments between health care needs versus social care needs, the subject of budgets and the allocation of resources all surfaced as key issues. There is a trend throughout Europe to substitute cheaper for more expensive services in an attempt to limit the costs of caring for an increasing elderly population (Baldock 1993).

Resources also appeared sometimes to be allocated inconsistently, demonstrating the need for procedures to be made available to clients and carers. Inconsistency gives the impression that resources are being allocated on a discretionary not a needs basis. Resource constraints are inevitable in a situation of finite resources but welfare decisions should still be reasoned and demonstrate equitable treatment (Coote 1992). The advocate's role, in all these instances, as perceived by the practitioners, was to maintain a person-centred approach whilst working to secure equitable treatment and resources that were appropriate to need, without becoming drawn into arguments over budgets. Advocacy would seem likely to assume increasing importance in the future as local authorities come under financial pressures and eligibility criteria are more tightly drawn.

MAINTAINING AN INDEPENDENT PERSPECTIVE

There were several instances in the study of clients being at the centre of major conflicts – between professionals, between a client and a carer, and between professionals and carers. In all cases the focus of the advocate was to ensure the client's voice was heard above the conflict and respected. Her independent status was seen by the practitioners involved as pivotal in unlocking the conflict. The carers, except in the case of client/carer conflict, appreciated the input of the advocate and perceived her independence as important.

In the one situation of client/carer conflict the advocate was unable to resolve the incompatibility of their differing needs but helped to shift the balance in the case, so that the client's voice became stronger, and the previously dominant influence of the carer diminished.

HELPING WITH DECISION-MAKING

Decision-making with dementia sufferers is clearly a source of anxiety for many practitioners. Norman (1987) has called for a shift away from a paternalistic, protective attitude towards an approach that explicitly contains an element of risk-taking and respects the rights of frail elderly people to self-determination. Practitioners in this study, as in the Stevenson and Parsloe (1993) study, expressed concern over what credence to give to statements by dementia sufferers, especially where their expressed wishes were at variance with their needs, and worried whether they understood the risks they were facing.

The advocate used a 'substituted judgement' approach: that is to say wherever possible she sought information about the person's past values and beliefs, as well as observing non-verbal behaviour, to gauge the person's preferences. The practitioners in the study perceived the advocate as using a different approach to themselves – one that they would have liked to emulate – but felt that the bureaucratic and time-consuming nature of their new tasks often forced them to adopt a 'best interests approach'.

THE LIMITS OF ADVOCACY

There was one case of financial abuse in this study, where the daughter was denying her mother access to her possessions and finances. The advocate attempted to mediate with the daughter, but when this failed it became necessary to secure legal representation to take matters further. The client had no estate to fund lengthy and costly legal processes and as none of the local solicitors had been willing to take on the case, the Legal Services Advocacy Project undertook the necessary work, in close co-operation with the advocate herself.

This particular case seems both to illustrate the limits of advocacy and the need for more flexible legislation. Research indicates that elder abuse is increasing, with financial abuse being a particular problem (Pritchard 1992; Wolf and Pillemer 1989). Cases of this kind offer support for the view of the English Law Commission (1991) that for advocacy schemes to flourish and develop they need the support of a 'firm but flexible legal framework' which could form part of a wider package of legislative reform (p.173).

In this context, it is interesting to note that the Scottish Law Commission (1993), recognising the deficiencies of the current legislation with regard to abuse of vulnerable adults, suggests that courts could have powers to grant exclusion orders where it appears that the conduct of another person is 'injurious to the physical or mental health of the (vulnerable) adult' (p.51). Advocates could play a vital role in such situations, by supporting the vulnerable adult and enabling their voice to be heard in the subsequent proceedings.

CONSEQUENCES OF ADVOCACY

The study suggests that advocacy is valued for its independent and more person-centred approach and ability to secure greater client participation and access to appropriate resources. It is also perceived by many practitioners as a different but complementary approach to decision making with dementia sufferers.

However, securing access to resources sometimes necessitated a challenge to health or social work service providers, and not surprisingly the advocate felt this resulted in greater defensiveness or hostility by providers as a consequence. Simons (1994) noted similar difficulties among service providers in adapting to the challenge of advocacy, and among advocates in establishing an accepted role.

Some key issues for the future

The UN Declaration on Rights of Disabled Persons elaborates an earlier declaration which incorporates the right to personal advocacy, and has been adopted by the United Kingdom. Despite this, and unlike other countries, the right to personal advocacy is not enshrined in law in Britain. Access cannot therefore be taken for granted, since there is no automatic right to the assistance of an advocate and some systems, notably hospitals, are less 'open' than others to their involvement (Ivers 1994, p.64). Consequently advocates may be denied access to their partners, to records and even to staff, and must be mindful that they have to deal with sensitive service systems which may not fully appreciate the advocate's role. Careful negotiation may therefore be called for to secure entry into the system.

Had the government implemented Sections 1 and 2 of the Disabled Persons Act, this would have provided an underpinning framework for advocates, which would have avoided many difficulties. This needs to be addressed for the future, either through legislation or, as Simons (1994) has suggested, a service users' charter, which would guarantee users the right to an advocate. Some hospitals are adopting this approach, but it is unclear whether this is a genuine wish to empower patients or more a desire to, 'offer token support and be seen to be fashionable' (Russell 1994, p.13).

Many advocacy schemes also suffer from two major drawbacks:

First, evaluation of their effectiveness is limited, and in some instances the partnerships appear to have more of a befriending role than an advocacy role (Carr 1990; Wertheimer 1993). Connor's (1993) study of project monitoring and evaluation stresses that their success is dependent upon clarity of project aims and workload. As funding authorities are placing greater emphasis upon evaluation, advocacy schemes seeking to secure funding will need to consider how they address this requirement for the future.

Second, funding for advocacy schemes is usually short term, making future development difficult. Where local authorities or health boards are the major funders then independence in the long term may be difficult to sustain (Ramcharan 1993), a problem exacerbated by the trend of local authorities and health providers towards formalising their relationships by the contracting process.

Not all models of advocacy, previously successful with other client groups, will necessarily transpose well to the field of dementia. For example, for self-advocacy to become a reality would require earlier diagnosis. Although GP's are reluctant to diagnose, the advent of memory clinics may be helpful here.

Citizen advocacy, with its emphasis on sole loyalty to the partner and on long-term relationships, may also not be ideally suited to a situation where one partner has a deteriorating illness and may lose the capacity to consent to the partner's activities. The question of trust, previously discussed, is very important but the issue of accountability would seem to merit further debate, as mere compliance with the advocate's activities *without proper understanding*, does not constitute informed consent (Clark forthcoming).

Despite these caveats, there has probably never been a greater need for advocacy – the new community care arrangements do not empower users, and carers as resources are allocated on a needs-led basis, with locally drawn eligibility criteria. The concept of clients as 'customers' is inherently flawed and criteria may become even more stringent as financial constraints increase and arguments between health and social care providers become more vociferous. Only the independent role of an advocate, focusing solely on the needs of the person with dementia, can ensure that they receive equitable treatment from service providers.

Concluding thoughts

Advocacy for people with dementia is assuming increasing importance as a consequence of the development of a mixed economy of care, changes in the health service and greater emphasis on cost control in service systems. These radical changes in the delivery of health and social care provide ample justification of the need for advocacy to ensure that dementia sufferers are placed at the heart of the decision-making process and that their voice is both heard and respected.

References

Age Concern England (1989) *Charters of Rights to Community Care for Older People.* London: Age Concern England.

Age Concern Scotland (1995) *Who Decides? Empowerment and Advocacy for Older People.* Edinburgh: Age Concern Scotland.

Allen, I., Hogg, D. and Peace, S. (1992) *Elderly People: Choice, Participation and Satisfaction.* London: Policy Studies Institute, pp.323–327.

Baldock, J. (1993) 'Patterns of change in the delivery of welfare in Europe', in P. Taylor–Gooby and R. Lawson (eds) *Markets and Managers: New Issues in the Delivery of Welfare.* Buckingham: Open University.

Baldwin, S. and Parker, G. (1988) 'The Griffiths report on community care.' *Social Policy Review 1988-89,* 143-165.

Barker, I. and Peck, E. (1987) *Power in Strange Places.* London: Good Practices in Mental Health.

Brandon, D. with Brandon, A. and Brandon, T. (1995) *Advocacy: Power to People with Disabilities.* Birmingham: Venture Press.

Broadley, E. (1990) 'Advocacy in a residential setting.' In M. Bernard and B. Glendinning (eds) *Advocacy, Consumerism and the Older Person.* Keele: University of Keele, pp.44–47.

Brownlie, J. (1991) *A Hidden Problem – Dementia Amongst Minority Ethnic Groups.* Stirling: University of Stirling, Dementia Services Development Centre.

Buchanan, A. and Brock, D. (1986) 'Deciding for others.' *Milbank Quarterly 64* (Suppl.2), 17-94.

Burton A. (1994) *Decision Making in Dementia: A Study of Advocacy with Dementia Sufferers.* University of Edinburgh, MSc thesis.

Bynoe, I. (1993) 'Rights and duties.' *Community Care,* Inside Supplement, 25 March.

Californian Department of Aging (1990) *Annual Report for California's Long Term Care Ombudsman Program 1988-89.* Sacramento, California: Californian Department of Aging.

Carr, S. (1990) 'The Development of Citizen Advocacy in the U.K.' Seminar paper at the World Advocacy Congress, quoted in Brandon (1995) p.97.

Carson, D. (1991) 'Clarifying the law on mental responsibility.' *Health Service Journal,* 16 May, 14-15.

Central Statistical Office (1991) *Social Trends 21.* London: HMSO.

Citizen's Charter (1991) *Raising the Standard.* London: HMSO.

Clark, C. *Paternalism, Citizenship and Community Care Policy.* Forthcoming.

Clark, C. (1996) 'Caring, costs and values: a concluding comment.' In C. Clark and I. Lapsley (eds) *Planning and Costing Community Care.* Research Highlights in Social Work 27. London: Jessica Kingsley Publishers.

Connor, A. (1993) *Monitoring and Evaluation Made Easy.* Edinburgh: HMSO.

Coote, A. (1992) 'Statutes of liberty.' *Social Work Today,* July 9th.

Counsel and Care (1991) *Not Such Private Places*. London: Counsel and Care.

Counsel and Care (1992) *What If They Hurt Themselves?* London: Counsel and Care.

Crawley, B. (1988) *The Growing Voice*. London: Values Into Action.

Department of Health and Social Security (1989) *Caring for People: Community Care in the Next Decade and Beyond*. London: HMSO.

Doyle, N. and Harding, T. (1992) 'Community care: applying procedural fairness.' In A. Coote (ed) *The Welfare of Citizens*. London: Rivers Oram Press.

Dunning, A. (1995) *Citizen Advocacy with Older People*. London: Centre for Policy on Ageing.

Dworkin, R. (1986) 'Autonomy and the demented self.' *Milbank Quarterly 64* (Suppl.2), 4-16.

Ellis, K. (1993) *Squaring the Circle: User and Carer Participation*. York: Joseph Rowntree Foundation.

English Law Commission (1991) *Mentally Incapacitated Adults and Decision Making: An Overview*. Consultation Paper No. 119. London: HMSO.

Fennell, G., Phillipson, C. and Evers, H. (1991) *The Sociology of Old Age*. Buckingham: Open University Press, pp.22–44.

Gilhooly, M. (1992) 'Proxy consent and the preservation of autonomy.' In *Consent to Treatment, Vol.1; Consent to Research, Vol.2*. Edinburgh: Scottish Action on Dementia, pp.26–34.

Gooby, P., Taylor and Lawson, R. (eds) (1993) *Markets and Managers: New Issues in the Delivery of Welfare*. Buckingham: Open University Press.

Greengross, S. (ed) (1986) *The Law and Vulnerable Elderly People*. London: Age Concern.

Henwood, M. (1995) *Making a Difference? Implementation of the Community Care Reforms Two Years On*. London: Nuffield Institute for Health/Kings Fund Institute.

Herr, S. (1989) 'Disabled clients, constituencies and counsel: representing persons with developmental disabilities.' *Milbank Quarterly 67*, Supplement 2, Part 2, 352-379.

Homer, A. and Gilleard, C. (1990) 'Abuse of elderly people by their carers.' *British Medical Journal 301*, 1359-1362.

Ivers, V. (1994) *Citizen Advocacy in Action: Working With Older People*. Stoke on Trent: Beth Johnson Foundation.

Law Society (1989) *Decision Making and Mental Incapacity: A Discussion Document*. London: The Law Society.

Marsh, P. and Fisher, M. (1992) *Good Intentions: Developing Partnership in Social Services*. York: Joseph Rowntree Foundation.

Marshall, M. (1986) 'Social work practice and private care.' In S. Etherington (ed) *Social Work and Citizenship*. Birmingham: BASW, pp.108–119.

McCreadie, R. (1989) 'Dementia and the law.' In *Rights, Risks and Responsibilities*. Edinburgh: Age Concern Scotland, pp.31–34 (Proceedings of Symposium)..

McGlone, F. (1992) *Disability and Dependency in Old Age: A Demographic and Social Audit.* London: Family Policy Studies Centre.

Mishra, R. (1990) *The Welfare State in Capitalist Society: Policies of Retrenchment and Maintenance in Europe, North America and Australia.* Hemel Hempstead: Harvester Wheatsheaf.

Moore, E., Connor, A., Martin, P. and Tibbitt, J. (1992) *The Hidden Safety Net: Mental Health Guardianship: Achievements and Limitations.* Edinburgh: Scottish Office Central Research Unit.

National Consumer Council (1990) *Consulting Consumers in the NHS: A Guideline Study.* London: National Consumer Council.

Neill, J. and Williams, J. (1992) *Leaving Hospital: A Study of Elderly People and their Discharge to Community Care.* London: National Institute for Social Work.

Norman, A. (1987) *Rights and Risks.* London: Centre for Policy on Ageing.

O'Brien, A. (1992) 'Who gets what, why, where, when and how?' *Generations Review* 2, 2, 16-18.

O'Brien, J. (1984) 'Building creative tension: the development of a citizen advocacy programme for people with mental handicap.' In B. Sang and J. O'Brien (eds) *Advocacy: The UK and American Experiences.* London: King's Fund Centre.

O'Hagan, M. (1993) 'Stopovers – on my way home from Mars', in *Survivors Speak Out.*

Penhale, B. (1991) 'Decision making and mental incapacity: practice issues for professionals.' *Practice 5, 3,* 186-195.

Phillipson, C. (1990) 'Approaches to advocacy.' In M. Bernard and B. Glendinning (eds) *Advocacy, Consumerism and the Older Person.* Keele: University of Keele.

Pritchard, J. (1992) *The Abuse of Elderly People.* London: Jessica Kingsley Publishers.

Ramcharan, P. (1993) 'Citizen advocacy for people with a learning disability in Wales.' In D. Robbins (ed) *Community Care: Findings from DHSS Funded Research, 1988-1992.* London: HMSO, pp.284–285.

Rankin, M. (1989) *Advocacy – A Case Study.* London: Volunteer Centre, UK

Russell, P. (1994) 'Still a bridge too far?' *Care Weekly,* February 3rd, p.13.

Scottish Action on Dementia (1988) *Dementia and the Law: The Challenge Ahead.* Edinburgh: Scottish Action on Dementia.

Scottish Action on Dementia (1992) *Advocacy for People with Dementia: Draft Discussion Paper.* Edinburgh.

Scottish Law Commission (1993) *Mentally Disordered and Vulnerable Adults: Public Authority Powers. Discussion Paper No. 96.* Edinburgh: HMSO.

Simons, K. (1994) *Citizen Advocacy: The Inside View.* Bristol: University of Bristol, Norah Fry Research Centre.

Social Services Inspectorate/Social Work Services Group (1991) *Care Management and Assessment: Practitioners' Guide.* London and Edinburgh: HMSO.

Stevenson, O. and Parsloe, P. (1993) *Community Care and Empowerment.* York: Joseph Rowntree Foundation.

Thornton, P. and Tozer, R. (1995) *Having a Say in Change: Older People and Community Care.* York: Community Care and Joseph Rowntree Foundation.

Tyne, A. (1992) 'Normalisation: from theory to practice.' In H. Brown and H. Smith (eds) *Normalisation: A Reader for the Nineties.* Tavistock/Routledge.

Wertheimer, A. (1993) *Speaking Out: Citizen Advocacy and Older People.* London: Centre for Policy on Ageing.

Wolf, R.S. and Pillemer, K.A. (1989) 'Helping elderly victims: the reality of elder abuse.' Quoted in C. McCreadie, *Elder Abuse: An Exploratory Study.* London: Age Concern and King's College Institute of Gerontology.

Wolfensberger, W. (1977) *A Balanced Multicomponent Advocacy/Protection Schema.* Toronto: Canadian Association for the Mentally Retarded.

Wolfensberger, W. (1983) *Reflections on the Status of Citizen Advocacy.* Toronto: National Institute on Mental Retardation.

Further Reading

Scottish Law Commission (1991) *Mentally Disabled Adults: Legal Arrangements for Managing their Welfare and Finances. Discussion Paper No.94.* Edinburgh: HMSO.

Sang, B. and O'Brien, J. (1984) *Advocacy: The UK and American Experiences.* London: King's Fund Centre.

The Contributors

Pamela Brown is a Research Officer, PSSRU, University of Kent.

Anne Burton is currently the manager of an assessment team for older people in Fife. She has previously worked in the field of mental health, drugs and alcohol abuse. Decision-making with mentally impaired adults has been a long-standing interest and formed the basis of her MSc thesis.

David Challis is Professor of Social Work and Community Care, PSSRU, School of Psychiatry and Behavioural Sciences, University of Manchester and University of Kent.

John Chesterman is a Research Fellow, PSSRU, University of Kent.

Murna Downs, PhD is currently Research Manager at the Dementia Services Development Centre at the University of Stirling. Her research interests include hospital resettlement for people with dementia and their care staff; care staff practices in long-stay residential settings; and general practitioners' approaches to the diagnosis and management of dementia.

Allan Gilloran, PhD is currently Senior Lecturer in Sociology and Social Policy in the Department of Management and Social Sciences at Queen Margaret College in Edinburgh. His previous research has focused upon staff work satisfaction and the quality of care in psychogeriatric wards in Scottish hospitals. He is presently working with Dr Murna Downs on a project investigating staff perceptions of, and reactions to, the relocation of people with dementia from a hospital to a residential environment.

Malcolm Goldsmith was a Research Fellow at the Dementia Services Development Centre and has recently published *Hearing the Voice of People with Dementia: Opportunities and Obstacles*. He is now involved in preparing training material based on his research. He is the Rector of St Cuthbert's Episcopal Church in Edinburgh.

David Gordon is Research and Development Manager with Lanarkshire Health Board. He has worked in both health and social care research, with a long-standing interest in elderly people and a particular interest in dementia.

Tony Holland is a University Lecturer in Developmental Psychiatry (Learning Disabilities) in the Section of Developmental Psychiatry of the Department of

Psychiatry, University of Cambridge, and Honorary Consultant Psychiatrist working in the Adult Learning Disabilities Service in Cambridge for the Lifespan Healthcare NHS Trust.

Susan Hunter is a lecturer in social work at the University of Edinburgh. She has a particular interest in the implications for vulnerable adults, including older people and their carers, of the recent changes in arrangements for community care.

Alan Jacques was for 17 years Consultant Psychiatrist at the Royal Victoria Hospital in Edinburgh and for the past two years has been a Medical Commissioner at the Mental Welfare Commission for Scotland. He has a particular interest in the care of people with dementia, and is Vice-Chairman of Alzheimer Scotland Action on Dementia and Chairman of the St Bernard's Club in Edinburgh.

Tom Kitwood is Senior Lecturer in Psychology at the University of Bradford, and Leader of Bradford Dementia Group. His present research is concerned with the social psychology surrounding the dementing process, and his work involves him in constant contact with persons who have dementia and their carers.

Mary Marshall is Director of the Dementia Services Development Centre at the University of Stirling. This centre exists to extend and improve services for people with dementia and their carers.

Gillian Parker is Nuffield Professor of Community Care and Director of the Nuffield Community Care Studies Unit, University of Leicester. Her main research interests are community care policy, informal care, disability and financial support for long-term care in old age.

Paul Spicker is Senior Lecturer in Social Policy at the University of Dundee. He has researched and taught a wide range of topics in social policy, including studies on poverty, housing, health and social care.

Richard von Abendorff is a Research Fellow, PSSRU, University of Kent.

Jill Warrington is a Senior Registrar in the psychiatry of old age currently working at Herdmanflat Hospital, Haddington. During a secondment to the Dementia Services Development Centre she prepared a literature review and practice guide for senior staff entitled *Depression and Dementia: Coexistence and Differentiation*.

Lawrence Whalley is a Consultant Psychiatrist and Crombie Ross Professor of Mental Health at the University of Aberdeen.